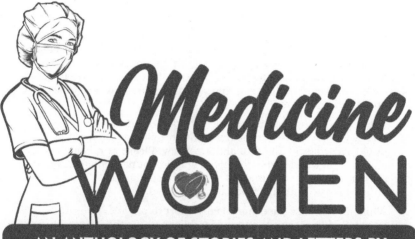

Medicine WOMEN

AN ANTHOLOGY OF STORIES AND LETTERS BY FEMALE DOCTORS AND HEALTH PROFESSIONALS

Dr Alisa Yocom	Kim Sheppard
Dr Ann Marie Balkanski	Dr Land Phan
Dr Anne Stark	Dr Melanie Underwood
Courtney Rickard	Dr Mokgohloe Tshabalala
Dr Erkeda DeRouen	Dr Olivia Ong
Dr Faye Jordan	Rebecca Lang
Helen Zahos	Dr Sana Jesudason
Dr Helena Rosengren	Dr Simone Watkins
Dr Jacinta Palise	Dr Talat Uppal
Dr Jessica George	Dr Vanessa Sammons

Compiled, edited, and published by CHANGE EMPIRE BOOKS

Published by Change Empire Books
www.changeempire.com

Edited & designed by Change Empire Books

While the authors have made every effort to provide accurate internet addresses at the time of publication, neither the publisher nor the authors assume any responsibility for errors or for changes that occur after publication. Furthermore, the publisher does not have any control over and does not assume any responsibility for author or third-party websites or their content.

Legal disclaimer:

This book is designed to provide information and motivation to our readers. It is sold with the understanding that the publisher is not engaged to render any type of psychological, legal, or any other kind of professional advice. The content of each article is the sole expression and opinion of its author, and not necessarily that of the publisher. No warranties or guarantees are expressed or implied by the publisher's choice to include any of the content in this volume. Neither the publisher nor the individual author(s) shall be liable for any physical, psychological, emotional, financial, or commercial damages, including, but not limited to, special, incidental, consequential or other damages. Our views and rights are the same: You are responsible for your own choices, actions, and results.

Authors have tried to recreate events, locales and conversations from their memories of them. In order to maintain their anonymity in some instances, authors have changed the names of individuals and places, and may have changed some identifying characteristics and details such as physical properties, occupations and places of residence.

LETTER FROM THE PUBLISHER

When a brilliant doctor I worked with on another book asked if she could take me to lunch, of course I said "Yes!" right away. Over a delicious meal she told me about a vision for a book, written entirely by female doctors.

"There are so many young women in medical school," she said, "but once you get into medicine, you realise how few women there are in leadership positions." She told me various stories about how women in medicine are subject to a lot of sexism, both from colleagues and patients alike, and there are regular comments about medicine and motherhood not mixing. "But it's hard for people to feel sorry for doctors," she added.

I loved the idea of the book, and although I had no doctors in my network, the word spread fast, and I was fortunate to bring together a group of incredible female doctors and health professionals to tell their stories.

During our coaching calls (try getting a group of 20 doctors and health professionals on a call at the same time!), I heard numerous stories which didn't make it into the final chapters – like the one about a gifted female surgeon walking into a pre-op consultation, only to be met with a patient asking, "Is a woman seriously going to operate on me?"

I don't know about you, but if I was getting surgery, I'd be honoured to have an accomplished, steady, caring woman performing the procedure.

I'll admit, I'd be the worst doctor in the world. I gag at the sight of a bruise, let alone blood! I volunteered for Radio Lollipop in my university years – a radio station in the children's hospital. I think I lasted two shifts. Being around children with cancer and other life-threatening conditions was more than I could bear, and I didn't even have children of my own back then. It takes a special person to do this day in and day out, and I'm so grateful to all the people in medicine who have this vocation.

Reading the stories in this book moved me to tears multiple times. The responsibility of caring for the lives of others and delivering difficult news, all while coping with sexism, stress, and challenges on the personal front, including illness, natural disasters, and strained relationships. Especially as a mother myself, reading how a doctor has had to tell a parent that their child is dying, or be there for a mother whose child has just passed, is something that I can't even fathom. The strength, compassion, and courage it takes to work in medicine is so far beyond what I feel I'm capable of, and I'm sure there are readers who will feel the same.

So, this book is about celebrating what it means to be a woman in medicine.

The woman who is a feminist, doctor, wife, teacher, mother, daughter, sister, friend, boss.

Be prepared to be moved by this book... to laugh, to cry, to be surprised and inspired.

I hope you enjoy Medicine Women.

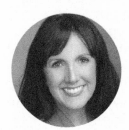

Cathryn Mora

Founder, Head Coach and Publishing Director
Change Empire Books

Instagram @change.empire.book.coaching
LinkedIn linkedin.com/in/cathryn-mora/
Email publisher@changeempire.com

CONTENTS

CHAPTER 1

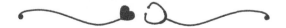

The storm before the silence

DR SANA JESUDASON
PAEDIATRIC REGISTRAR

"Now, I don't mean to be offensive, but..."

I groan inwardly. We're at breakfast, and I'm just about to attack a scandalously high stack of pancakes. We're one of three couples sharing this table, lining our stomachs before getting classily wasted at this afternoon's wine tasting, and the speaker is our hostess. She's just finished a questionable rant about immigrants, during which I have wisely hidden behind my foot-high flapjack tower. As a tiny, sassy lady-doctor of colour, it's a line I've heard more times than I can count: "I don't mean to be racist/sexist/offensive buuuuuuuuuuttt TADAAAAAAAA!"

I brace for impact. My scathing inner jackass fights the urge to pigeonhole her, but she's just spent half an hour lamenting the fact that "they just need to learn to speak the language," and then, espying the sole person of colour at the table, tried to rapidly backtrack by complimenting me on "how good my English is". Oh, and her name is Khelsee, which sounds like a name she made up because, presumably, Kelsey wasn't interesting enough. Ohhhhh, Khelsee, I'm trying, but good Lord, the pigeons doth swarm!

"I don't mean to be offensive, but you doctors just make way too much money! I mean, caaaah-monn, there are so many other people that work just as hard as you do, am I right?"

1

I shoot a quick look at my partner, who is suddenly very interested in his toast. As far as offensive statements go, this one is actually fairly benign. I smile with blithe grace and make a self-deprecating joke about orthopaedic surgeons and golf. It's a smile that Mona Lisa would be proud of, so little does it betray the scornful, petty asshole that lurks beneath. It's a paediatrician smile.

"Yes, I know you don't want us to vaccinate your baby, but Vitamin K is...a vitamin." Smile.

"I understand you're refusing antibiotics for your septic child because you're afraid of lead poisoning..." Smile.

"So, you make your son drink his own urine for good health? Alrighty, then." Smile.

The older I get, the more I hate this about myself: I am a textbook people-pleaser, a chronic self-deprecator, an insufferable milquetoast. My mother carefully raised this doormat to never offend, to always comply, to submit, to smooth over. It is who she is, and who I am. It is this version of myself who cracks joke after joke after joke after joke when I'm being insulted. It is this person who bends over backwards to diffuse tension that I did not create. So hyperextended is her spine, she could practically kiss her own ass, and LORDY wouldn't her mother be proud *(don't say ass, kannama, it's not nice)*.

Unfortunately, my mother also accidentally raised a tiny sweary ragemonster with a strong sense of tribal justice. The casual rudeness of our friend Khelsee rankles me in a way that it usually wouldn't. She doesn't know me. She doesn't know who I am or what I do. She doesn't know what I've seen. I recognize my own hypocrisy with a start; haven't I just done the same thing? Come on, Sana. Maybe she really is "afraid" and not just racist. Maybe she really is a mumpreneur, not just a lady who paints mugs that no one asked for. Maybe she contains fucking multitudes, I don't know.

The difference is, I have the common courtesy and self-awareness not to blurt these mean little thoughts out loud. I mean, is it ever acceptable to confront a complete stranger about their income? Did I fall asleep and wake up on another planet where the rules of polite conversation don't apply? Should I start telling her what I think of Jesus and the Labour Party and eugenics? Should I show her my rash?

I'm well aware of my petulance. I mean, it's a silly thing to say to a stranger, sure, but I'm not someone who gets upset easily. Any other week, I would brush it off, thank my lucky stars that I get paid well to do something I love, build a bridge and get over it. But not this week. Not today. Not after my last shift in the ED.

***

The Emergency Department is a cacophonous clusterfuck of activity. It is a whirling dervish of screamed instructions, ignored orders, bleeps, blips and sirens, blood, guts, and raw fear. I've always marvelled at it: a place where a furious mother screeches that you're ignoring Jaydynn's severe papercut, while in the next bay, a little old lady stoically bleeds to death because she "didn't want to disturb anyone." Shining fortitude alongside whining pique. Lives are saved, bones are mended, hearts are restarted, and entitled malcontents with their vaguely sore toes are quietly ignored until they leave in a huff.

That is not what it looks like now.

"SHUT UP, everyone, it's an arrested baby."

The nursing team leader holds up an angry hand in the universal gesture of SHUSH. The rest of the nonsense falls away; there is suddenly nothing more critical than this phone call.

She starts scribbling furiously on a progress note, shorthand demographics that cause every heart in the room to sink further and further with each qualifier. 9moF. 8kg. Known cardiac pre-op. Found unresponsive. Cyanosed. 40 minutes CPR. Unknown downtime. Intraosseous access. Oxygen saturation unrecordable. I can almost hear the hope drain from the room.

We take comfort, cold as it is, in the mundane busywork of getting ready. We pace around the room, drawing up drugs, sourcing bags of fluid, preparing an intubation trolley. Someone makes sure we've paged anaesthetics. Another calls the paediatric ICU to reserve a bed. We write biometrics, drug doses, tube sizes on the board. Maybe if we reduce the fear into a pat little set of figures and pictures and neat trolleys, we can trap it in a box.

The resus bay is silent, tense.

3

The paramedics arrive. They bring the baby across to a comically large bed, never breaking their CPR. Their calm, professional handovers betray a silent desperation. We've all worked in paediatric hospitals for years. You'd think we'd be used to this by now.

We're not.

I stand, a dumbass deer in the headlights of blinding competence. In my view, everyone in this room is the pinnacle of medicine: take the hardest thing you do, and make it smaller. This is the most exquisite of timepieces, the most intricate of Rube-Goldberg machines, the most flawless of executions in the face of impossibly high stakes. Everyone has a job, everyone does it well, and everyone is trying so, so hard. So hard.

In the blur of urgent orders (could someone order an X-ray we're going to give a fluid bolus has someone called cardio fuck we lost the IO have we considered bicarb WE NEED ACCESS), I overhear a poor junior who's picked the unenviable task of taking the history. The baby's mother is incredibly calm. She looks younger than me.

She tells us that the baby is supposed to have surgery next week to fix her heart. She tells us she fed really well that afternoon. She tells us she's started saying "mama", that she's growing beautifully, that her cardiologist is really happy with her, that she's starting to cruise on furniture. She tells us a thousand little stories that she desperately needs to share with someone, anyone, as if she can turn back time by the sheer magic of folklore. Someone gently asks her if she started CPR at home, and her answer shatters the air with the force of a bullet: "I tried, but I guess I didn't do a very good job, haha!"

Oh, lord almighty, that laugh. I fancy myself a wordsmith, but I will never have words for how horrifying that mirthless little giggle was. The icy, naked terror spilling out of her and roaring through the room like an arctic gale. It is one of the most awful noises I've ever heard. I didn't know it then, but that dubious honour would be snatched not once, but twice more in the next hour.

We've been going for about 50 minutes, and I've stepped up in a plastic gown to take over CPR. I have a horrible sense of how springy this chest wall is; nothing like the brittle snappiness of adult ribs, breaking under the mandated force. We will restart your heart at the expense of your broken body, and don't you bloody forget it.

The baby is a shade of indigo that barely belongs in nature, let alone in humanity.

The circulation nurse puts the kindest, gentlest hand on my shoulder and whispers, "I think we're stopping, doc."

We've run through so many cycles of CPR, so many rounds of adrenaline, so many treatment algorithms, and then...it's over. The ED consultant asks over the din if anyone has any objections to us stopping CPR, because there is truly nothing left. It's a moment overflowing with mercy. She unearths the agonizing truth that we've all been too afraid to vocalize, buried under layers of heroic effort and hypercompetence. We've all known this was coming from the first line of the handover, but we wouldn't be in this field if we didn't believe in, and hadn't seen, undeniable miracles. We wouldn't be in this field if we didn't hope, just a little. She expects, and receives, no challenge.

I take my hands off the chest and step down off the stool they've thoughtfully brought in for us, the vertically challenged resuscitators. We all stare at the monitor, transfixed. We know what's coming, but there's a familiar combination of panic, nausea, and despair that starts in my belly and rises, rises, rises, pausing along the way to stab me in the heart, rattle around in my ribcage, and snake a hand around my throat. We hear the droning, unbroken scream of the telemetry alarm: GUYS, THE HEART'S STOPPED, WHAT THE HELL ARE YOU DOING! As if any of us needed the aural confirmation of what we had just done. The technicolour visual was more than enough, thank you.

And then, silence.

Imagine sitting in a boat in the centre of a calm, still pond. You lay back, a straw boater covering your face, and bask in the sunshine. The gorgeous freedom. The casual innocence. The simple, exquisite pleasure of weightlessness. Perhaps the smell of a world freshly washed after rain. Now, imagine your lungs are filling with water. You try to scream, but there's no sound. You try to swim to the surface, but your limbs are lead. Your lungs are lead. The water is lead. You are drowning, drowning, drowning, and no one is coming to save you.

That is what this silence feels like. Chilling. Perverse. Like none of us will make it out of here alive.

The silence is punctured by a soft thwack, and my peripheral vision registers movement. An experienced nurse has stepped forward and caught the mother in her arms, as she collapses into the awkward embrace. We all turn to watch, wordless. A howl emanates from her lungs, the sound of a chasm opening deep within her, ripping through her, amplified by the suspended animation of the resus bay.

I'm not certain if you've ever heard the cry of a mother who's just lost her child.

Yes, there is the all-encompassing anguish. Yes, there is a black hole of agony and unimaginable, palpable loss. But that's never the note that stands out most to me.

It's the incredulity. It's the brutal decimation of the belief that bad things don't happen to children. It's the sound of the death of innocence.

It's the rending of a soul, railing against this most unnatural of horrors: a child dying before their parents.

It's a Molotov cocktail through the window of a church, because if she ever believed in God, she most certainly doesn't any more.

Her cry breaks the spell. Suddenly, the world reanimates, like someone has pressed play and turned up the volume. The bustle resumes; someone takes the leads off the baby, another half-walks, half-carries the mother to the bedspace, another makes note of the time of death, another starts to quietly clear the room. Another, her face ashen, runs to grab the warmest bunny rugs she can find, a task as desperately urgent as it is unnecessary. The same cacophonous clusterfuck, but muted. Attuned. Respectful. It's a tacit acknowledgement that right now, everyone's problems are trivial bullshit; if you have never watched your baby arrest and die, you are not welcome in this moment.

We watch her propel herself forward, the loneliest woman in the world, on the saddest, most interminable pilgrimage of her life. For a second, she can't locate her baby's arm for the giant stupid bed and the slithering mass of cables. In this moment, I hate myself, oh, I hate myself. I am filled with a shame and loathing so powerful, so very irrational, that we have subjected her to this final crushing indignity. She is all alone, and we've just made her scramble through piles of worthless tubing to find this tiny, cold, blue hand. A tiny, cold, blue hand that we couldn't save.

So, you see, Khelsee.

I'm well aware that I make money. It's good money, too. It's good enough money that I feel guilty about it, vaguely ashamed of it. It doesn't feel fair that my work should fill my soul this much and make my heart beat this fast, but also manage to feed my body and pay my rent and satisfy my gluttonous need for shoes and pocket dresses and miniature tea sets. I've heard and awkwardly laughed at every hilarious yacht-related joke at my expense, a simultaneously humanizing and dehumanizing us versus them. The lazy orthopaedic surgeon/anaesthetist/dermatologist teeing off in tremendously stupid pants and one glove, while the good, hardworking, blue collar folk tarry on, clad in sackcloth and pathos. It helps when you think of us as an amorphous field of tall poppies, smugly sauntering off towards a necessary beheading. It helps when you don't think of us as people. People who get divorced a lot, who commit suicide a lot, whose parents die and whose kids have soccer games and whose wives go into labour, all while we're trying like hell to help a total stranger whose needs just happen to be more immediate (and they always, always are). No, never mind them.

Never mind the lonely, terrified intern weeping quietly in the hallway, pulling their eleventh unsupported 9pm finish in a row. Never mind the brilliant female surgeon, sexually harassed and then summarily fired by her mentor for daring to complain. Never mind the desperately unhappy anaesthetic trainee, quietly, surreptitiously pocketing leftover propofol/insulin/morphine, with a deadly precision and expertise.

Never mind the 27-year-old girlwomen who watch children die, and then come back to work the next day full of foolish hope that we'll help the next one.

Don't get me wrong, Khels. I absolutely love my job. Many of us do, and sometimes, that love is the only thing you have left.

But there is an irreversible heaviness, a leaden poison that settles within our hearts. It's the feel of cold, blue hands, it's the sound that hope makes when it dies, it's the stupid Harry Styles song that your 12-year-old neuro patient played 47 times a day (the song that played at her funeral). It's the haunting that feeds the insomnia. It's the list of names that I can never use for my own kids, because they're irretrievably, inextricably suffused with pain.

I don't think the point, as you eloquently put it, is that "I make too much money."

The point is this:

Someone has to bear witness to these ghosts. Someone has to willingly submit to being haunted their whole lives, to periodically, shamefully googling their names to reread their obituaries, to holding holding holding it together, only to weep in quiet corners of different hospitals six months later. To being a little emotionally unavailable to the people that we know (hope) will forgive us; our husbands kids sisters mothers. To becoming progressively less raw and soft and progressively harder and darker, all the while maintaining an outwardly sunny disposition (this is paediatrics, after all).

Someone has to carry all this damn baggage, forever.

Now.

Is there any amount of money that I could pay you to do that for me?

And would it ever, ever be enough?

I didn't think so.

CHAPTER 2

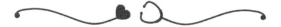

Path of most resistance

DR VANESSA SAMMONS
NEUROSURGEON, PERIPHERAL NERVE SURGEON

When it's over, I don't want to feel like I didn't taste it. I want to feel part of life and to acknowledge my contribution.

Like any intense relationship, neurosurgery has given me a lot. I have had so many rich experiences; some of them are good, and some of them are bad. I don't regret *most* of the scars on my heart; when I think of the episodes that put them there, I realise the appreciation for life and all of its experiences that my scars augment. Neurosurgery has also taken from me: it has taken my time, it has caused me to lose friends, it has taken my patience for the world that exists outside of the hospital – where I control so much of what happens and when. Has it made me a nicer person? Sometimes I would say yes, and sometimes I would say no.

Tonight, as I sit on the cool sand in the fading light of a challenging day, I am thinking – maybe too much. Tonight is a supermoon. I know a lot about supermoons because I have a daughter who is like me in almost every way, and she likes to tell me everything she learns about space and all that is out there, way bigger than us, and bigger than anything we can imagine. The light this rare moon casts over the harbour is simply spectacular. I watch the light reflecting off the ripples on the water and wonder how big this expanse would be if there were a ripple for every human on the planet. That thought makes me feel small; it makes me feel like I am insignificant, and that the things I do on this planet don't matter. This is in stark contrast to how I so often feel: like every little action and decision I make is enormous.

My mind went to that Wednesday, which was just one little Wednesday in an ocean of Wednesdays. My pager made its sound, the one I loved for the experiences it gave me but hated for the same. I was not in the operating theatre, and I had seen all of my patients, so the rest of my day was spent responding. Responding to calls from the ward, responding from consults and calls from other specialties, and, with this particular call, responding to the trauma page.

The rush of words came: "A man in his forties, hit in the head by some metal beam on a building site. Big gash on his head; I can see bone and there is significant blood loss. He's intubated. When the ambos arrived he was unconscious, GCS 3, right pupil fixed and dilated."

I remember the contrasting feelings of excitement and dread. I was relatively junior, only one week into my second year of doing this; this case sounded difficult, and it was as much of a neurosurgical emergency as it gets. I called my boss, grateful for who was on call that day.

"Vanessa, you've got this. Clean it up, extend the incision as you need to, remove the blood, find the bone fragments, and close up. Expect to extend the craniotomy around whatever the injury is, and when you close it, leave the bone flap out."

My still-hot-coffee abandoned, I hurried to the trauma bay. My heart rate would have increased anyway with the speed of my walk, but the very real but unreal experience had my heart rate well above whatever the walk would have achieved.

There was an intense internal confusion that occured: *I am young and inexperienced. I can't really fix someone who has been injured so badly that their skull is fractured.* Yet, there was a total awareness of the task ahead, and I sank into a deep focus. I am aware these days, in situations like this, of how my peripheral vision seems to disappear and I somehow become aware only of the sounds that I am meant to hear. I am good in a crisis – and this was a crisis.

As I was scrubbing for the case that Wednesday, I paced up and down in the small scrub bay, running through what my steps would be, imagining what I might encounter and how I might deal with it. I was aware of my heart beating, but I was also aware of how in control I felt.

There was a nasty skull fracture: a piece of skull – a part of the body that should never touch the outside world – was stuck vertically up into the air. Underneath, I found the dura, the lining around the brain, was torn, and I could see the injured brain. Lucky, I thought at the time, this was right frontal. Lucky indeed. There is the contrast again. Was this man very lucky or very unlucky? If there was an expendable part of the brain, this was it. If the injury was concentrated here, this man could be okay. I did my best. I did what my boss suggested – and tonight, as I replay it all in my mind, sitting here on the sand under the bright supermoon, I know there is nothing I could, or should, have done differently.

That thought, the thought of having done it right, made my mind search for a contrast. With actions, it's often clear whether you have done the right thing, but words are more complicated. I wonder what the moon was like on the night I spoke the words that made someone realise their world was changed forever.

***

The corridors were quiet and the lights were dim, which was usual for this part of the hospital, where patients often stayed for a long time and the emergencies that brought people and action happened slightly less often. As I walked alone, I reminded myself, again, that I had to stop wearing these shoes; there was something about the soles, maybe the rubber or the pattern, or maybe the shape, that squeaked loudly and irritatingly with every step. Somehow the sound I made when I walked felt like an insult to the reverence I needed for what I was about to do. I took a seat at the computer and opened the viewer that allowed me to look at Michaela's scans once again. I had just gone through it with my boss, so I had the heart-breaking image etched in my mind – but there were no mistakes allowed here. I reminded myself of the level of the fracture, T12/L1. It was at the junction of the thoracic and lumbar parts of the spine. I was much more used to looking at CT scans and seeing the squares of each vertebrae stacked one on top of the other in a gentle curve. But not this time. The fracture was immediately evident, and the discomfort I had felt earlier in the pit of my stomach returned. She was 23 and had been in the middle seat when her friend failed to see that the car in front of them had stopped, ready to turn right. Michaela hadn't noticed the intense pain initially, she said, but she did notice that she couldn't quite tell where her legs were. She felt safe when she was finally removed from the car by the paramedics, and everyone in the hospital had seemed so in control. In the spinal ward, the nurses were all so kind, and the place had a more homey feel than other parts of the hospital, so when I went to her bedside and stood near her mum with my bundle of paperwork, I was greeted with another one of her grateful smiles. Grateful for the pain relief she now had. Grateful she was alive and well cared for. And grateful that she was going to be okay. But she wasn't really going to be *okay*, not in her previous understanding of that word, and that was the purpose of this evening's visit.

I suddenly became very self-conscious. Did I look like someone she could take seriously? How were my clothes today? Did I look put together, in control, sensible and capable? My stupid shoes. I stood there and felt very tall next to her completely reclined body. Should I sit? No, she wouldn't be able to see me as well given that her young eyes were facing the ceiling.

"Hi, Michaela." I tried to meet her smile but second-guessed myself. "I am here to talk about your surgery tomorrow and do the paperwork."

"I need surgery?" she asked.

"Yes. Michaela, you have some bones in your spine that are broken and we need to line things up again and keep everything in place with some screws and rods."

She nodded, thus far unperturbed. The nod hurt, because it told me she was not aware of the gravity of her situation. I looked at Michaela's mum and knew instantly that she was, most definitely, aware. The look of despair on her face contrasted with a look of incredible strength as she focussed on her child's face.

I explained to Michaela and her mother, a broken woman of strength, about the surgery and the things that can go wrong, trying to sound like I hadn't said it many times, trying for it not to sound like a string of words falling out of my mouth without any conscious thought.

12

"Now, Michaela," I said, "you need to know what to expect after surgery, assuming none of those complications happen." An earnest nod. "The purpose of the surgery is to stabilise the broken bones to allow you to sit up. That way, you will be able to participate in rehab sooner than if we were to leave the bones to heal on their own. The surgery will decompress the bottom of the spinal cord, but it won't make it work again." I stopped. What else could I say here?

I saw a flicker of confusion, and then panic.

"What do you mean?" She paused, eyes wide. Her next words were faster and slightly louder. "Am I going to be able to walk again?"

I knew the answer was no, but that word felt so blunt, so definite, so final.

"I don't think so," was all I could manage.

Michaela's left hand reached for her mum and she began sobbing and calling out. "Mum, Mum, Mummm."

My own breath became shallow and sharp, and I found I couldn't swallow. This was the first time I had told someone that they would never walk again. It wasn't about me – but had I done it the right way? Was there a right way? Were my words right? I will never be sure, but that evening will continue to pop into my head for the rest of my life.

Tonight, sitting on the sand, I still wonder how, and how much, she really remembers. I wonder where Michaela is now. She would be nearly 35 years old. She will never know that sometimes I think about her and tears still well in my eyes.

A few tears escape my blinking eyes and roll down my cheeks as I rub my bare feet into the sand, looking for some kind of comfort. I think about the tiny volume of water that forms a tear as I look at the expanse of water in front of me. I realise, at this point, that I'm a little cold. Cold is a strange sensation. When you aren't cold, you can't imagine being cold, and you certainly can't remember or appreciate just how horrible it can be. It's only when you're already in it that you realise how much you want to be out of that state.

It's empathy, I think, that helps you to understand the things people do when faced with various situations or feelings. The

13

funny part is that how people act can be vastly different – even contrasting – on any given day. What governs that? Most of the time we will never know; perhaps most of the time the person doesn't even know.

There were days when I was in training, simultaneously loving and hating what I was learning, days where I looked forward to getting a page or a call, and other days where the shrill tone of the pager needed to be silenced. On the days I needed silence, I would flick the switch and the sound was replaced by a violent vibration. So violent that if the little black box were on a table, it would vibrate itself to the edge and leap into the abyss. Which was exactly what happened on the day I treated my first gunshot injury. I had once met a colleague who was doing their neurosurgery training in Detroit. He saw a gunshot wound most weeks, which is something I still fail to comprehend. *Was he exaggerating just to be cool?*

On this particular day, I scrambled to pick the little thing up off the floor so I could see who I had to call back. I knew the number instantly; it was one that used to fill me simultaneously with excitement and apprehension: the trauma bay.

"28 year old male. He was GCS 4: moving his right arm and leg before being intubated. He's got a bullet in his brain."

I said I was on my way, and within a minute, I was looking at a very peaceful patient on a ventilator in the trauma bay. It was a confusing sight. There was no blood, and his head and face all looked intact. "Self-inflicted" was what the emergency doctor told me; I noticed a small injury on his neck, on the right, just below his jaw. The scan was on the screen of the nearby computer. I scrolled through the unbelievable images and realised that it was highly likely he would survive. There was very little bleeding within the brain; the bullet had entered the skull and magically avoided all of the major blood vessels in the head, and there, just below the top of his skull, was the white, irregular disturbance on the scan that represented the bullet.

Now, on the beach, at night, seems a world away from the operating room that day, even though I can still picture it perfectly. We are normally animated and communicative, much like a sports team, all working together to get it done. On that day, there was silence and a kind of communal disbelief and sadness. We weren't brought together by someone having done something wrong to this patient; we weren't feeling the usual unity that occurred when someone was in an accident or had an illness, when we are all aware that it could have been any one of us. This was different. We were all trying to understand what had led to this moment for this young man. We assumed we were doing the right thing, but there was a moment *(was it a long moment or a short moment?)* where this man wanted a completely opposite outcome to what we were trying to achieve, *for him.*

I mechanically removed a small window of bone just above where the bullet had rested and used forceps to pick the bullet up and remove it from the patient's frontal lobe. There was a weird clink as I dropped the distorted metal object into the clear plastic jar being held out to me. I put a small tube into the fluid space within the brain so we could monitor his intracranial pressure, just in case the damage was more severe than at first thought. His operation was relatively minor and uneventful, which felt completely out of keeping with what had occurred.

The tube was removed after a few days, when it was clear that his brain was not going to swell dangerously, as it can after a trauma. This man would never be the same, however; he was left with weakness on the left side of his body, and his cognitive function and personality also changed, but how much I'll never know. I wonder how he processed what he did to himself and how he manages in life now. Maybe he lives with an intense feeling of joy wrapped in intense sadness, trying to make sense of experiencing both at once, realising that in order to be dead, he had to entirely give up being alive.

I am often aware that our choices, by their very nature, mandate giving something up. I sit here on the sand, in the cold, alone and looking at the moon. It means I am not in my home, warm, with my children, smiling and laughing. I wonder about my choices and what I have given up. A slight feeling of anger makes my face feel hot, even though my half-buried feet are still cold. I have tried many times to erase some memories, but memories can be hard to erase, even more so when emotions are connected to them.

"Why are you even here? Why are you bothering?" Silence.

"Why don't you just go and be a mum?"

More silence.

The room was already cold, like operating theatres almost always are, but these words felt chilling. This person was my boss, entrusted with teaching me how to be the best neurosurgeon I could be. Those words felt threatening and were said with a wry smile that I could feel rather than see because of the masks we were both wearing.

Concentrating on the feeling of the sand between my toes, I try to focus on where I am. This night is simply beautiful, and the reflection of the light across the water is trying its best to help me maintain a sense of peace. Try as I might to sit in insignificance on this beach, on this planet, in this solar system, in this universe, I can still see my boss's large shape, made bigger by the surgical gown, standing across the operating table from me. I remember people in the corner chatting, oblivious to what was being said in the centre of the room, beneath the bright lights. The anaesthetic machine kept the beat as air was pushed in and out of the patient's lungs; the patient's heart rate was an audible rhythm. My hands were steady, but I had to concentrate on keeping them so. They held instruments that were millimetres from a patient's spinal cord. *What a tiny distance a millimetre is in the context of space.* There was a job to do, and I had to keep doing it. I couldn't engage and I couldn't escape. Could anyone else hear this? Would they say anything if they did?

I had just returned to work after having my first child during my specialist training. In my naivety, I imagined that this would make me somehow more impressive. I am a woman, training to become a neurosurgeon, and I was a mother. Here I was, trying to do it all and giving it my all. I simply never imagined that motherhood could give the impression that I was not dedicated to my chosen profession; I didn't know that I would be considered by many to not be worth teaching.

Training to become a neurosurgeon is six years of physically and mentally gruelling work. When you are offered a coveted place on the training program, you think you have done the hard part. *I am going to be a neurosurgeon*, you tell yourself, almost with an air of disbelief. But disbelief comes with the realisation, over and over during years of training, that many of those who are meant to be teaching you this craft have no interest in actually doing so, and perhaps might even take some perverse pleasure in making you fail.

Recently, a surgical colleague was describing an international colleague to me. In his words, "She is one of those people you love to hate." He went on to describe her career, how successful she was, how wonderful her work life seemed to be, and how nice she was. "You really want to hate her," he said, "but you sort of just can't."

I genuinely like people I admire or people who are impressive. How many people think this way, and how often can people control their desire to dislike people for their successes? The targets of bullies are usually those who are successful or have traits that the bully secretly admires or covets. The profile of the bully target includes those who are competent, well-liked and self-assured, and a threat to the perpetrator; they are people who have a desire to help, heal, teach, and nurture. They are also typically fair, honest, and ethical; they have integrity. Can bullies not realise that even people they despise for their perceived perfection have their *things? Everyone has things.*

At age seven, I became the child of an only parent when my father was killed in a car accident. Over the years, I have reflected on the impact this has had on my character and my decision making. I have become a person who wants to do everything. I want to experience it all, and I don't want to leave this world without making an impression. I suppose things could have gone the opposite way. Who knows? I could die tomorrow, so why bother trying too hard? Why bother putting myself through pain? Why bother fighting?

But that isn't what happened to me. I want to do it all now, while I am here, and I can. My biggest problem in life is that some things are mutually exclusive. It is simply not possible for me to be a neurosurgeon as well as a paediatrician working in poorest Africa. I would love to be a high court judge shaping society through my thoughts and decisions. I watch our political world, often with distaste, and wonder how I would embrace altering our human world if I were leading a country. I would have loved to be a prima ballerina. I have this perhaps arrogant self-belief that I could have been any of those things, and I would have done them well. But here I am: a brain surgeon. When I say it out loud, it sounds wacky, impossible, fanciful. Is that even a real job, or is it something concocted to enable jokes?

As a medical student, I found neurosurgery, or it found me. Quite honestly, it appealed to me because it seemed like the hardest thing to do. The knowledge and skills required, the hurdles one has to jump to be selected...and, of course, it's fascinating. Like a stoic mare, on went my blinkers, and neurosurgery it was going to be. I still think that choosing the thing that seemed the hardest was far too facile a way to choose a career. I never really contemplated what it would mean and how I would be affected. Even if I had, I expect it would be much like trying to imagine being cold when I am not, or like now, warm when I am not.

I am happy here on the beach, with only the sound of the waves, because I need a break from people and being assessed, sized up, judged, no matter how positive any result may be.

"What do you do?"

"I'm a doctor."

"Oh, a general practitioner?"

"No, a surgeon."

"Oh. What area?"

"I am a neurosurgeon."

"Oh. Wow!"

Steps backward, eyebrows raised. Eyes dart from my face to my toes and to the top of my head. I have just been totally re-evaluated. Many people don't know what to say next, and it's awkward. I wonder if it is uncomfortable for everyone, or just me, because I have seen it over and over again, this same flash of confusion and surprise. I am looking for it, waiting for it, and when people take the information in their stride, I can't help but wonder, perhaps arrogantly, if they genuinely aren't surprised or whether there is an effort to hide it.

Being an unexpected neurosurgeon is socially awkward, and I don't know whether it's me or them. I don't look like the stereotype, and when the conversation occurs, it's confusing. As time passes, I am becoming accustomed to the profound impact my work has on every aspect of my life. Most importantly, I am learning to be authentic within it. I no longer try to give people what I think they expect from their neurosurgeon. Instead, I give them me, the girl who also likes to walk on the beach when the moon appears, to ponder the universe and all we don't know, to think about all the things I am, and have, and all the things I have given up.

Several years and many craniotomies later, I think about the man across the operating table, my then boss, who was trying to make me feel like I didn't belong in this special group of doctors, making me feel like I didn't have skills, like I didn't have something to bring to this coveted society; he was telling me I should leave and "just be a mum." He wanted me to fail – was it for sport?

But I didn't fail, and at the end of an operating day, as a consultant neurosurgeon, I inevitably reflect on the day and think about how I have impacted someone else's life. Occasionally, I also reflect on the training I endured to become what I am, and the life experiences that have shaped me. I think about people who want to see failure or feel threatened by another human's success and thus treat them with disdain. I think about the occasional people who didn't want to contribute to my success because of what I now see as their own personal failing, and I say, *"thank you for the compliment."*

As I walk on the soft sand back home, cold but content, I understand that I will probably continue choosing the path of most resistance in life because, to me, this is what life is…a series of incredible adventures, where the heart is broken and put back together time and time again but will forever show the scars.

CHAPTER 3

Someone like you

COURTNEY RICKARD
MEDICAL STUDENT, MICROBIOLOGIST, NURSE

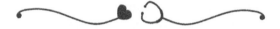

"Someone like you, someone with a trauma history?"

Why did she say that?

Is she trying to casually drop a diagnosis on me that everyone but me can see? Could I really have somehow missed that the not-so-great parts of my history were not-so-great enough that they fall into a "category"?

I'm not ready to be in a category. It's so distracting that she keeps speaking while I'm trying to hide my astonishment. I keep what I hope is a neutral expression on my face as I decide where to shelve this until I have time to unpack it.

If I have to be in a category, then I'd like to be in the "No, I'm fine; look at all the things I have" category. She must not realise. Can't she see that I'm successful, not broken?

My mind, so adept in having an answer to every question, is racing. My opposing responses are immediately ready and internally firing back at her like a rapid-fire machine gun, shooting out my defensive answers from every direction. Fortunately, or unfortunately, depending on your perspective, I recognise that I am having a physiological stress response. The hallmarks are there, just as the medical textbooks describe. My heart is racing, my mouth is dry, and it's fight or flight time

When Walter Cannon described his "fight or flight" nervous system response theory in 1915, he was referring to wild animals exposed to a predator; but in this century, his theory has been adapted to include modern day threats, like a dodgy driver, preparing to give a presentation to your class, or an off-the-cuff innocent utterance from a professional who clearly assumes you have evaluated the significance of your own past.

The prevalence of lions, or other primal threats, might have been more common-place when Walter was researching his theory, but as I look around now, there's not a lion in sight. I'm guessing that if I fight, try to fly off, or even play dead, then this will not end in a way I'll be pleased with.

Mine is a wired-in response. My neurological pathways have been reinforced by repeatedly being sent into this emotional state. Akin to a gym enthusiast building a bicep by using heavy weights, causing repeated trauma. My trauma muscles are mighty. I've unknowingly become better at diffusing this over the years, but rewiring requires repetitive positive experiences.

I remember many of the not-so-great wiring experiences with all of my senses.

Running down the hallway to the relative safety of my childhood bedroom is a regular occurrence. Somehow, it allows me the time to weigh up that, whilst my tiny feet would get me there faster than his, I might not have time to close the door and jam it shut with my cupboard door. A perfect architectural design flaw that keeps the monster out.

Searing hate in his eyes, enough to shrink a child into a crumb. Thin lips and yellowed teeth hurtling spit as he yells to assert his dominance. His aggression, like an ocean swell trying to swallow me, is followed by the chaos of tumbling inside a wave until it disperses its force and recedes from the damage without a care for the destruction it leaves in its wake.

Blood turns into ice in this moment, or so it feels, as he tries to slide something under the bedroom door to remove the trusty cupboard-door safety device. But it isn't my blood that freezes;

it is my ability to love myself and my future successes that he is freezing.

When the violence has passed and quiet blanketed my space, I believe the threat had melted away. I'm not tall enough for the exciting rides at theme parks yet; I have no hope at this age of comprehending that he is wiring me to expect and accept this in my future.

The lion will one day be gone, but the wounds will remain.

Healing will happen most of the time. Young, healthy bodies do a wonderful job of this. Children are fabulous, pudgy bundles of stem cells, newness, and hope, often requiring a mere hug to overcome an owie and return to conquering their day. One problem, though, is that not all wounds are visible and not everybody has a healer or a hugger to help.

I always wanted to help.

These healers and huggers are magical people. My family doctor, a healer – people keep calling him a GP – is clearly a wizard. Assisted by his equally magical nurse. Masters of owie fixing.

I want to help.

These are my people.

This is the future I want.

I might only be fun-sized right now, but I know this feels like the path I should follow.

My pre-school teacher was astonished that I could read, even more so that I told her about cumulonimbus clouds. So excited was my spongey little brain to absorb all that the world had to teach that I would fall asleep reading nature guides, stories, and day-dreaming of all the wondrous things I could do if I were bigger.

The bigger I was, the more the disappointment stung when I failed to unleash my amazing in the way they'd all hoped.

"Such a shame. She has so much potential."

There was, in fact, an awfully large effort being made, just in the wrong places. The effort required to hide the truth of a stepfather's shortcomings is immense. A veritable shopping list of cover stories, lies, and emotions to suppress. The world will surely explode if people find out. If I am as dreadful of a child as he says, then it's clearly best that nobody else realises.

Thankfully, my grandmother never realised. Thankfully, she was a hugger. A woman and a gift at the same time. Somehow warm sunshine had been packed into this tiny, bouncy, kind-hearted soul. She danced through her days wearing a smile that felt like holidays and giving out hugs that felt like calm safety. A true dynamo who always saw the positives, despite the challenges.

The crutch provided by her love was an irreplaceable aid in my arduous climb to adulthood, and a reminder to never give up. The monsters can't retain their apex-predator position forever. The only way they win is if we choose to inherit the dysfunction and become the next monster.

But I will never do that. I will not pass on his anger and hatred. I want to love and nurture. I want to heal and hug. I want to help.

I may have been diminished to a glacial pace, but progress is progress, and sometimes surviving is the progress we need to make in that moment. I do exactly that. I become an expert at covering and squashing down the emotional injury. I focus on putting one foot in front of the other.

His presence, a chain around my ankle, but I was born to fly upwards, so this can't always be the way.

Although I temporarily escaped the savage for the safety of another country, there came a time when I returned to the house, fuelled with the youthful arrogance of being close to my twentieth year. Surely, he can't try to hurt me now.

I am wrong, again.

I hear the distinct clinking of metal as he retrieves a knife. I know this fight needs to stop.

This moment is different. This needs to be thrive, not survive. Some flames are harder to extinguish than others, and a mere flicker can cause an explosion. He was right. They were right. So much potential has already been wasted.

The familiar process of a rushed analysis of the situation feels like effort that I know I am no longer prepared to keep making. Nearest lockable door, tick. Does it have an exit on the other side, tick. But I'm an adult now, and he isn't worth this expenditure of energy. He just isn't worth missing out on my future anymore; I've missed out on so much.

The excuse making, the cover story creation, "being strong and pushing through" – it is a grueling and all-consuming task. For a child, it seems like the weight of this task is crippling, and it was.

As a woman, it is a task I am no longer prepared to take on.

A deadlock has been installed on my bedroom door; it will take him a few minutes before he tries to go around and enter from the other door. As the phone rings, I prepare my final threat to my mother. It's very simple; her future only has one of us in it. There are teams now, and there's one chance to join mine.

I want to help. You need to let me.

As I jump off the balcony and sneak out of the yard to the freedom of the street, I know this is a pivot point. Memories of powerlessness steel my resolve. The sounds of the ceramic vase smashing and screams echo in mind as I recall him dragging a child half his size down a hallway. Her long, usually perfect hair whips around in the chaos as she tries to break her ankle free of his grip. I couldn't help her then, but I can do this now.

Did you know you can spell freedom with three letters? DVO.

He's gone.

There's much grey in the distinction between naivety and hopefulness. I am both naive and hopeful.

Time to breathe, and live, and evolve.

Ready to fulfil my desire to help, I dip a toe in the waters of the industry that feels like home. My nursing application is submitted. Laced with hope but peppered with doubt.

Where does the wasted potential go? Can I get it back? Is too much of it gone? Was he right?

This is the wound festering. A microscopic cut growing into a thriving, contaminated ache.

Microbiology is a fascinating subject. 10,000 E. Coli partying hard in a space smaller than a pinhead, evading our human eyes but nonetheless there, and absolutely able to cause catastrophe at their whim. An entire world, existing inside another.

Emotional wounds exist this way. Unseen, partying away in dark corners of the minds of innocent victims. Chewing up self-belief and wreaking non-specific damage to avoid detection. Not everything needs to be seen to be real or be felt. Confidence can be amputated like a limb.

At my glacial pace, I continue. Qualifying for my nursing license, the metaphorical foundations for my house of safety.

In the presence of the wonderous souls known as health care workers, I continue.

I want to help. I love to help. Each nursing shift rebuilds a piece of my worth. These patients think I'm helping them, but every shift that passes I grow happier and healthier and stronger. These are the repeated positive experiences needed to rewire from the trauma.

My spark of curiosity flickers.

I am grateful for the opportunities I've been entrusted with, to comfort others through frightening times. My nursing uniform, a symbol to them that they don't need to know my name to know they're safe and that I will advocate. The gravity of holding the hand of another as they exhale and leave this world; there are no words for this. These moments transform you. The peaceful exit of a soul who is prepared and trusting.

The hospital is a little different tonight. Hurried, disorganised and lacking its usual well-oiled-machine vibe which usually makes a day feel more like a choreographed dance. I respond to the call for anyone up-to-date on their work to help return the turbulence to tranquil. As I enter the room, I see the eyes of a soul who is not ready to leave. He is being taken. Unwilling, unprepared. His arm hangs over the bedrail; he was mid-escape as he started to lose this battle.

Waiting for an emergency team to arrive feels like an eternity as we lose him. Absolute silence as we wait for a heartbeat that never arrives. The chaos is unnoticeable. Cords, tubes, machines. Fluid all over the floor, and a room of disbelieving people who want to help because he's too young to go.

Screams from his wife, lashing into my depths as the doctor changes her existence with one sentence.

She didn't see this coming. She trusted our uniformed delegation but we're not always afforded an opportunity to change an outcome.

Could I have done better? Been faster? Would he have been safer if another nurse walked into that room?

It's the middle of the night. His tearful son led to a room to absorb the prospect of life without daddy. Without his fearless leader. Without his hero. Without a goodbye.

I want to help more. I want to help bigger. I want to help better.

I'm wired to believe that I can't, that I'm not worthy, but at my glacial pace, I continue.

I collect degrees and knowledge, but my dream isn't satisfied. I conquer things that I'm told are "beyond" me. I buy property as a single woman, I learn to ride a motorbike, I travel, and I try to be loved, but I haven't undone all of the damage. I expect that I'm deserving of another monster, and he finds his way to me.

I feel the metaphorical chain lock around my ankle again as this new monster threatens to tear our life apart should I be so ridiculous as to chase my medical career dreams.

The knocks seem to do more damage when you've been here before. The familiarity of the fear. Knowing the level of internal fortitude required to climb out of the mess, and the uncertainty of wondering how to start again.

My car is blocked by his ute, with intent.

My keys, confiscated.

The path to the exit has him between it and me. This is what I'm worthy of. Confirmed by the police as I arrive at the station, to be told that taking his keys and driving his car to the safety of the police station would allow him to charge me. I'm unworthy of their protection because I have no evidence to show that he threatened my life.

I arrive trapped in the cabin with him standing in the ute tray because I locked the door before he could grab me. I can't understand why this doesn't indicate that he is unstable, or that I am in danger. But again, I am wrong.

My grandmother would say, "Oh well, it's water under the bridge." I know somehow I owe her memory a debt of gratitude, so at my glacial pace, I continue.

We were five siblings and now we are three. I mourn for the lost futures of the two who chose to extinguish their own flames but I can't choose this path for myself. Pivot, survive, thrive and breathe.

Everything has a price, but some rewards are unexpectedly fulfilling. The fear of starting over, alone and unsupported, was immense. The satisfaction of following my heart and being free of volatility is invaluable.

I will follow my own path now. Medicine was waiting for me all along.

I existed too scared to apply for the opportunity to have the fulfilling days I was born to experience. Potentially older, potentially wiser, but still full of potential.

Degrees in hand, lump in throat, and heart pounding. My medical school interview is complete and the universe takes over where the monster left. Some potential had hidden itself well enough to escape my past and hold my hand into the future.

They hadn't realised I wasn't supposed to be here by the end of my first year. The imposter syndrome, a fading relic of days gone by.

As I finish my medical degree, and as I find my place in the world, I know I am exactly where I am meant to be. So excited to help. So grateful for the opportunity to do so. So in awe of my remarkable, altruistic colleagues. So far from perpetuating the hate.

I am generous. I am kind. I am a motorbike rider, a nurse, a microbiologist. I am an MBA qualified businesswoman, a friend, and a lover of jewellery and nice cars. I have a family, a future, and hope. I am many things, defined only by myself.

And I am ready to delight in spending my days as the doctor I've worked so hard to become.

CHAPTER 4

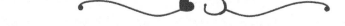

DR HELENA ROSENGREN
SKIN CANCER DOCTOR AND EDUCATOR

"Don't move or you'll die!" my father calls.

Arms extended, he leaps confidently from the boulder beneath his feet. He flies over my mother, who is crouching on a rocky outcrop at the water's edge, gutting freshly caught fish. The brilliant sunlight dances on the surface of the water, seaweed silently swaying back and forth beneath it. The ocean laps softly against the shoreline, and the boat we moored just twenty minutes earlier rocks gently close by.

My mother laments the generous splash of seawater that envelops her as my father hits the surface. "Oh no! I only just washed my hair this morning!"

My brothers and I start laughing uproariously. All five of us – Lars (14), Erik (10), myself (8), Sven (5), and our baby brother, Karl (15 months) – sit in a row against the wall of a cliff edge behind my parents, warming ourselves in the glorious afternoon sunshine. We have just jumped off the boat for an invigorating swim in the cool waters of the Kattegat Sea on the west coast of Sweden. It is a perfect summer day.

My father floats back up to the surface of the water, which suddenly blushes crimson around his head. Our laughter stops abruptly. A distant seagull gives a shrill cry and I taste the sea salt on my lips as I watch, with bated breath, waiting for my father to move. But he just floats there, face down in the water. As the seconds drag past, I become aware of the brutal pounding in my tightening chest.

Lars suddenly springs into action, navigating the rocks to jump into the water. He turns my father over so that he can breathe and floats him back to where my mother is crouched. She cradles his head, body still in the water. He is motionless, and blood pumps from a gash on his right temple.

"Quick, kids – go and get help!" she shouts desperately.

We are on a tiny, rocky island in the middle of the ocean, having spent the day boating and exploring other remote islands. Curiously, my father, who usually goes out of his way to seek isolation for his family, chose to land where there are other holiday makers. Admittedly, we found our own little private bay, but we saw other families on either side of the headlands as we pulled in.

My heart thumps faster as I feel the panic rise within me. Erik starts to scramble over the rocks to the adjacent bay on our right. Little Sven, wide-eyed and pale, breathes fast and furiously beside me. I have the desperate urge to wrap him up and take him far away from the disturbing scene that has unfolded so shockingly before us.

"Come on!"

We start running as fast as our little legs can take us, up the track on our left and over the headland. "Help, help!" we call out as we climb down into the next bay.

"It's our dad – he dived into the water and he's not moving!" I shout.

"There's blood everywhere," adds Sven.

A man gets up straight away and quickly strides towards us. His little boy, who like me must be about 8 years old, runs after him.

We hurry back over the headland with our helpers in tow. However, the sight of my father's motionless body below us as we round the corner stops us in our tracks. Dazed, I stare down into our little bay, where two men are struggling to lift my father's limp body into their own boat. Lars has climbed into their boat and is helping, too. As they all struggle to lift my father aboard, the little boy beside me asks, "Is he dead, Pappa?"

His father prods him and puts a finger to his lips. "Shhh."

Eventually, they get my father aboard the vessel. Lars stays in the boat with the owner, and after some hurried words with my mother on the shoreline, the motor starts and they whizz off towards the mainland and the closest hospital. She stares after them, struggling to hide her fear. For the first time, I notice an unknown lady holding my baby brother Karl. She is talking to him softly, pointing the other way to save him from seeing the horror of what we have just witnessed.

Sven and I quickly climb back down into our little bay. The shocked onlookers wander away, shaking their heads in disbelief.

Meanwhile the other gentleman, who has so kindly come to assist my family, offers to take us back to our holiday rental cottage on the mainland in our own boat and is helping to gather up our things. Instilled with a doctrine to leave nature the way she found it, my ghostly pale mother is trying to wash clean the blood-stained rocks where she held my father's head. I rush to help her, bewildered at the sight of my own father's blood.

We return to our simple dwelling, the cottage we have rented for the summer holidays. Once back, we sit and wait an eternity for Lars to return home and report whether my father still lives. My mother tells us to pray that my father will survive this terrible accident. I plead silently, desperately, with a God in whom I passionately believe, as I rock back and forth: "Please, please let Pappa live." I repeat it over and over again. I have already promised my God that when I grow up I will be a nun and don't know what else I can barter now in exchange for my father's life. So I just remind him of my promise.

Fragile and trembling, my mother makes us a simple evening meal, which she herself leaves untouched. After many hours, the police finally return Lars to us. He confirms without preamble that our father is dead.

"The doctor said that Pappa must have died at once from a broken neck when he hit his head on a spike of rock that he couldn't see under all that seaweed."

Our worst fears brutally confirmed, the tears now flow freely. It is impossible to comprehend that we will never see my father again. How could this strong, powerful man be taken from us so abruptly and so completely?

Much later, gathering her strength as she wipes the tears from her eyes, my mother explains to Lars that, as the oldest, he must let my grandparents know that their only child has died. My mother can't drive and my grandparents have no phone at their country home. The quickest way to get this tragic news to them is to send Lars in person. He is to make the six-hour trip to Stockholm by train at first light, then travel by bus out to their country cottage.

The family is in limbo, shocked and fragile, as we wait and wait for Lars to return. He takes much longer than the expected two days, and there is no way of checking in with him or my grandparents to make sure he got there safely. Much of the time my mother just lies in bed, silent and ashen white, getting up only to make food for us. We play quiet games in the garden, trying not to disturb her as we endlessly wait for something to happen.

Towards the end of the third day, her brow furrowed and face tight with anxiety, my mother walks to the cottage down the track with a request to use their phone to alert police that Lars has not returned as expected. I hear the police officer gently reassuring her: "He's had a terrible shock and he's probably gone somewhere quiet to take it all in. Or maybe he is just visiting a friend." The whole village has heard of our plight, and the kind neighbour suggests a friend who will be able to drive us all to Stockholm in our car on Lars' return. My mother welcomes this solution. Ever practical, it is Erik who now packs up our family belongings and helps prepare for our departure while I keep the little boys happy and occupied.

I wonder what will become of us. My father has played a pivotal role in the family, and a life without him is totally unimaginable. Until now, the longest I have lived anywhere is seven months, because my family is continually on the move. We have tended to drive south down through Europe after the long Swedish winter, once the snow melts and it warms up again. The car literally became our home as we searched for a week or two for our new summer holiday home, which was often in a small coastal village in Spain or Italy.

I recall how my father would dress smartly in a crisp, white shirt to go to work and would usually be away for a few days at a time. After my mother had finished home-schooling us, we were free to explore the glorious countryside. Frequently, the family would go to a remote, deserted beach or a mountain stream, where my brothers, father, and I spent long days swimming and fishing. Meanwhile, my mother tended to the baby and ensured food was ready for the next meal. In the evenings, the whole family would gather to play our favourite card games. We came home to Sweden in the winter, when we would rent a house and go to school for a few months somewhere near Stockholm, so that we could be close to my grandparents.

Apart from my grandparents, my parents seemed to know no-one. My older brothers and I made fleeting friends during the months that we attended different schools. The strict family rules were, however, that we could not visit or invite anyone outside school hours.

This is only the second summer since I was born that we have stayed in Sweden. And this is the first year ever, much to my delight, that my father planned for the family to return to the same rental property and schools after the summer holidays. I am so looking forward to seeing my very best friend again.

"When are we going back to our real house?" I gingerly ask my mother. Tears well up in my eyes when she replies with a tired voice that we are never going back and that we will instead be moving to England! Seeing how upset I am, she promises that when she finds us a new home, we will be settling down and going to the same schools for years to come.

On the fifth day following my father's death, we are overcome with relief when Lars finally reappears. "Sorry it's taken so long, but I boarded a train going in the wrong direction and it took me a whole day to figure out that I was travelling further and further north," he says quietly, cheeks flushed pink.

My grandparents have kindly offered to house us in Stockholm for the time being while my mother decides what she will do. They have two small units four doors apart in a smart apartment block in the city centre. Oddly, when not at their country cottage, they live relatively separate lives in each of their units, though my grandmother brings in meals throughout the day for my grandfather. Once back in Stockholm, my mother and the three younger siblings take up residence in the smaller unit, while my two older brothers make themselves at home in the larger one.

My father's body reached Stockholm a few days before us and on our arrival, my mother goes to see him. Afterwards, she tells me, in hushed tones, how surprised she is that, even though he has died, his hair and nails have continued to grow.

"Can I go and see Pappa too, please?" I ask, but she responds that children are not allowed to go to funeral parlours or to funerals.

A few days later, my father is buried following a desperately sad, lonely service, attended only by my mother and grandparents. In the weeks that follow, our family takes the underground every Sunday to visit the vast, beautifully maintained cemetery. It's a long, peaceful walk down cool, tree-lined gravel pathways. When we get there, I help my mother cut and arrange the fresh flowers we have brought. I try, unsuccessfully, not to imagine my handsome, injured father lying quietly in a large wooden box a few feet below me.

On one occasion, my grandmother comes with us. Tears streaming down her face, she hugs the simple gravestone. "I miss you so much, my son, and I pray every day that I will soon be with you."

My cheeks wet with tears, I feel unspeakably sad, knowing that there is no way of consoling her.

Apart from the weekly trip to the graveside and the odd visit from my grieving grandmother, I'm left looking after my two younger brothers every day during the long weeks following my father's death. Meanwhile, my mother packs up our rental home outside Stockholm and attends to all the official paperwork with solicitors, bank managers, and my father's employer on her own. My older brothers, having endured strict paternal parenting all their lives, have gone somewhat off the rails and are enjoying their newfound freedom.

Sometimes I beg my mother to let us accompany her back to our previous rental property to help pack up.

"We would be so good, Mamma," I say. "I'll keep the boys quiet and I'll help you with the packing, too."

"No, Helena. You are such a wonderful help here and I'm getting everything done so much faster this way. I don't know what I would do without you."

Placated, I take care of my little brothers as best I can. I change nappies for baby Karl, read the only book we have, a children's Bible, to Sven, and feed us all at lunchtime. My days are long and boring, but I'm glad of the company of my brothers and delight in assisting Sven to learn to read certain words. We fill our days giving baby Karl simple commands: "Open the door... Fetch my shoe... Put the book on the table..." and are amazed that he can follow our instructions. He, in turn, smiling widely, pleased with so much attention, gladly plays along.

At times, Sven and I talk about our father and wonder if his spirit is with us in the room right now. My father stares sternly at us from his photo frame, making direct, unblinking eye contact. Wherever we sit in the little unit, we cannot hide from his unforgiving gaze, but we do not dare turn the photo around. In life, he had often been playful, especially with us younger children, but the photo that remains is a stark reminder of how strict and disapproving he could also be.

When I get the chance, I talk privately to my grandmother about the planned emigration to England, which is really concerning me. In hushed tones, she tells me that my mother has family in England, with whom she will no doubt be making contact. Suddenly I ignite with excitement and curiosity. This intriguing family secret is a complete revelation to me! I didn't even know that my mother is not a native Swede. I probe my grandmother for more details, but she doesn't seem to know any specifics. Intuitively, I know not to question my mother to learn more. Nonetheless, the prospect of relocating to England suddenly seems so much more appealing.

Finally, what has seemed like an eternity to me is over. It has been six weeks since my father died, and we are ready to embark on our new lives. With most of our belongings now in storage, my mother and two older brothers will be responsible for three medium-sized suitcases. Little Sven is to carry a satchel with a few toys. My job will be to keep baby Karl safe. On the evening of our departure, our grandparents wave us off at the train station. Though close to tears, they also seem relieved that we are moving on, allowing them to have their units back for the autumn.

We journey south through Sweden and Denmark and the next day catch the overnight ferry to Harwich, England. That evening, feeling very tired after another couple of train journeys, we finally alight at the sleepy riverside town of Kings Lynn on the east coast of England. My mother has told us that our new home will be here. She promises that we will soon have proper beds to sleep in, as she heads to a hotel across the road. Sadly, there are no vacancies, so we keep walking. After visiting another three hotels, it becomes apparent that everywhere is booked out with holiday makers.

Weary from so much travel, my feet scrape along the pavement as I carry baby Karl, who refuses to walk. It is now completely dark, and we find ourselves by the river, where we sit down together on a couple of park benches. The air is warm and the rhythmic sound of the water close by is very peaceful. The whole town is turning in. Soon the twinkling lights from the homes behind us are extinguished one by one. Yawning and heavy-eyed, we lean against each other. Karl lies down on my lap and soon we are all sleeping soundly.

I wake to gruff, deep voices. Two police officers have shaken my mother awake and are asking questions, pointing at us all. I cannot understand the conversation, but it is clear to me that they are wondering why we are not sleeping comfortably in beds.

"This is ridiculous," my mother says to us quietly. "He doesn't believe you are my children!"

Lars, who seems to understand English well, speaks up to defend my mother, but his foreign accent does nothing to allay their suspicions. My mother finds our passports (five Swedish and one English), all bearing the same surname, but this does nothing to convince them. She pulls out my father's death certificate, but as this is written in Swedish, they shake their heads in bemusement. They confer quietly and next thing, wide-eyed, our hearts thumping, we are up and walking again with our heavy loads as they usher us along the silent back streets.

Finally, we find ourselves at a police station, where the six of us are locked in a police cell for the night. Exhausted, I finally fall asleep again, comforted that at least we are still all together. In the morning, Inspector Heaven cordially explains that he will send my mother's official-looking paperwork off for translation to see if her story can be verified. He looks doubtful that this will be the case. My mother whispers to us all, "Behave normally with me. They seem to think I've falsified your passports and abducted you all..."

We are allowed out of the cell but have to stay in the police station. Two young policewomen smile broadly at the sight of small children and pull out some toys, pens, and paper for us. I play happily with my brothers, feeling safe and secure with my mother in sight. Sometimes I catch the police officers giving her furtive sideways glances, shaking their heads in seeming disbelief.

In the late afternoon, Inspector Heaven, looking exasperated, tells my mother that the translation will not be available till several days later as a photocopy has been sent off to Sweden by ordinary mail. He would like to make an arrest and involve child services but has the sense not to be too impulsive. An hour later, a police van drops us all off at a local bed and breakfast. The owners' welcome is disdainful at the sight of this dishevelled, apparently unlawful group of refugees that have not washed for a few days. My mother is under strict instructions not to try to run and to check in at the police station every morning and afternoon. She is mortified.

"What an appalling welcome to my own home country after a tragic bereavement. They should be ashamed!"

It ends up taking five days for the translation to make its way back to the police station. We present as usual in the afternoon to meet a red-faced Inspector Heaven.

"I have to apologise," he says. "I should have believed you. You have acted very bravely."

The very next day, my mother's plans to settle here having been shattered by unwanted police attention, we head south again by train. Now realising the folly of arriving late, she has us settled in a caravan at the campsite in Clacton that afternoon.

After a couple of weeks in the caravan, we relocate to a rented three-bedroom home in the little seaside town of Frinton-on-Sea. Fortunately, my mother is now receiving a small widow's pension organised by an international organisation in Sweden, where my father had been employed. He was so confident that he would always be able to provide for his growing family that he had not thought to set up life insurance. Concerned about our family's predicament, the people in charge have miraculously managed to organise a small pension. So, we are reasonably comfortable, with my mother able to afford school uniforms, rent, and modest food.

After the flurry of activity since my father's death, my mother welcomes the quieter times with four of her children suddenly at school. She is sad and listless a lot of the time, so every day I help care for my younger brothers, prepare meals, and do whatever I can to try to bring a smile to her face. I'm also enjoying school and the challenge of learning English and am grateful for my mother's interest in this.

Ten weeks after my father's death, my ninth birthday comes and goes without much mention and certainly no presents. Both my older brothers and my mother also have birthdays that go by unnoticed within three months of his death. Two months later, Christmas is looming. In Sweden, we always had joyous celebrations at Christmas. My mother used to cook and bake for weeks ahead, make festive decorations with us, and ensure that everyone received a present from everyone else. This year, she does not have the will or the strength to even acknowledge Christmas. Wanting to give my little brothers at least some semblance of normality, I rescue decorations made at school, make cards for everyone, and paint rocks to give them as presents.

Some more months pass and I forget all about my Swedish grandmother telling me of a secret English family. One day, however, seemingly out of the blue, my mother informs us that we will be seeing our English grandmother very soon! As the oldest, Lars meets her at the train station after her five-hour trip from Bath, carries her luggage, and walks the short distance back home with her. My mother has instructed us to stay in the kitchen and come individually to the living room after our grandmother arrives, so that she can introduce us one at a time, from oldest to youngest.

When the front door opens, we stand listening silently behind the kitchen door as our mother quietly greets her own mother at the front door and then introduces Lars, her oldest son. They go through to the lounge and then Erik, with his warm, engaging smile, is ushered in and presented. Karl, unable to contain his excitement any longer, scrambles out of the kitchen and rushes into the lounge room to see what is going on. Not quite two years old, he is cute as a cherub with blond, curly locks. I let Sven go next as he is visibly put out that Karl has somehow managed to push in ahead of him. By the time I am introduced to my diminutive grandmother, she is seated and shaking violently, tears welling up in her eyes. Seeing my concern, she says simply, with a faint Scottish accent, "Hello dear, don't worry about the shaking. I'm just a wee bit surprised by all this. It's Parkinson's and not usually so bad."

I nod quietly, understanding that this must be quite a shock. In the space of a few minutes, she has suddenly acquired five grandchildren that she clearly had no idea even existed.

It also transpires that I have two lovely aunties and a boy cousin about my age. We witness a joyous reunion between my mother and her sisters when we meet them a couple of weeks later.

(Fast forward eight years to when I am 17.)

Though the facts remain hazy, I have come to understand that my father disapproved of my mother's family and insisted on an absolute separation. Through the powerful healing bonds of the women, our family is now firmly reunited.

Every summer, my Swedish grandparents come to spend a few weeks with us. Raw grief over the loss of their only child is never far away, but they are delighted to have become acquainted with my mother's family. When Lars and Erik completed their schooling, we all moved to Bristol to be closer to my extended English family. I have grown very close to my Scottish grandmother and both my aunties.

It is my Scottish grandmother who has instilled in me what a privilege it is to have an education. She has always encouraged me to study hard and do the very best possible academically. She grew up in Glasgow, where she had to look after her ailing mother from a young age. However, this did not deter her from getting an education. Extraordinarily clever, she would diligently study her school textbooks and complete all assignments brought home for her by two brothers, who could still go to school. She went on to study at Glasgow University in the evenings, where she chose to specialise in ancient Greek.

Her family was left virtually penniless when their father died suddenly. Her two brothers had left school, but with the depression of the 1930s looming, they were unable to find employment. My grandmother embraced secretarial training and then was lucky enough to be employed full time despite the Great Depression. From the age of 20, it was she alone who provided financial support for her whole family during this international crisis. Spurred on by the love of learning, she used her lunch breaks to learn Greek verbs, always maintaining her position at the top of the university class.

I am saddened that despite my grandmother having such drive and ambition, she was never able to aspire to a career in her field of interest. She would dearly have loved to have become a deaconess, assisting in church ministry. She tells me women in the 1920s were rarely able to fulfil their dreams and that I am lucky to have been born into a different era. Inspired by her story, I decided when I was only 10, that, no matter what, I would be going to university one day, making the most of the opportunities offered by modern education. It is now time to commit to that university degree.

"Whatever you do, Helena, make sure you don't study just for the love of it," my mother advises. "Go for a career-based university degree so that you can always provide for your own family, come what may. Look at me. I majored in double degrees in Spanish and French. When I first qualified, I was mortified that the only work I could get was in a department store. So, I went on to do an MA in French in Paris, which is where I met your father. The rest of course is history. As you know, despite now being registered with many translation agencies to try to supplement our meagre Swedish pension, the opportunities for work are few and far between."

Having seriously toyed with the idea of becoming an architect, I decide instead to apply for electronic engineering. Ever supportive, my mother and grandmother are very pleased with my choice of such a male-dominated career. I apply for a scholarship and am offered one by British Aerospace. I go on to attend interviews at three different universities, where I also meet engineering students and get shown around the campus. And each time, I go back home feeling a little depressed and totally uninspired by my career choice.

At the fourth interview in Sheffield, I meet an enthusiastic young electronic engineering student who tells me about a research project she is doing with childless couples who are contemplating test tube baby pregnancies. For the first time, I feel excitement stir as I listen to her. On the train journey home, it strikes me, like a bolt of lightning, that my enthusiasm was sparked because she was dealing with real people in crisis rather than electronic circuits. And just like that, in a split second, I decide I will become a doctor!

Until that moment, Medicine as a career choice has simply not occurred to me, as I have not studied the right subjects at school. Sharing my mother's love of languages, I chose to study German instead of Biology three years ago; and Biology is an essential prerequisite for medical school. Undeterred, I decide now that I will be doing another year at school to complete a Biology O level and also a Chemistry A level, another hitherto unachieved necessity for medical school. If my grandmother could push through despite the challenges, then so can I.

As I ponder my future more deeply, I realise that Medicine will be an ideal career choice for me. I love helping others, and the sight of blood or sickness has never been a deterrent. Having grown up with four testosterone-pumped brothers, injuries in our household are quite commonplace. "Helena, he's bleeding! Can you sort it please?" my mother will frequently call out, looking slightly green, with eyes tightly shut. She loves recounting how, at the age of 3, I sat for days outside my parents' bedroom in Sicily while my father lay sick in bed with rheumatic fever. I was waiting for him to stir so that I could cool his brow or bring a glass of water. When I was 4, he yelped in pain after accidentally stepping on a sea urchin in the Canaries. I was the only one he would allow to gently pull the painful spines from his fleshy, tender sole.

I remember my father frequently sitting me on his lap and saying, "My little Gullgumma, you will be so wonderful at looking after Pappa when he grows old." As a youngster I never took this seriously, but my mother has since confirmed that his intention was absolutely for me to care for him into old age. Had he lived, I would never have had the opportunity for higher education or a career without breaking ties with my family. Heartbroken though I have been all these years to have lost him, I also realise that the second before he decided to make that fateful dive was a sliding door moment with the power to change the entire course of all our lives.

41

Little do I know how challenging and deeply rewarding my decision to become a doctor will be as the years unfold. I know nothing yet of the long hours of study, into the early hours of the morning, that will be required as a medical student and later as a doctor pursuing a career in general practice and subsequently skin cancer medicine. I am oblivious of the intense working conditions of my first years after qualifying, when I will toil 70 to 120 exhausting hours a week caring for sick and dying patients as I upskill in various areas of medicine. I am blissfully unaware that one day I will move continents and shoulder the financial and emotional responsibility of caring for my own children, far away from the support of my extended family, while also pursuing a career. The personal sacrifices, exhaustion, and the immense sense of achievement of having opened and run a much-needed community-based skin cancer clinic for well over a decade has yet to unfold. The joy, passion, and satisfaction involved in research work, writing papers for publication, lecturing, and training other doctors is also something I will be privileged to experience.

And if I knew these things, as I sit on the train contemplating my future, aged 17, would I still embark on this journey or choose a different pathway? I am a shy and unassuming teenager and would not believe myself capable of fulfilling this charter. Perhaps it is just as well that I am oblivious to the dedication and focus that will be required for the decades ahead.

CHAPTER 5

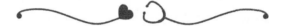

DR JESSICA GEORGE
GENERAL PRACTICE REGISTRAR

Dear Tanya,

I wish that when we had first met as 9-year-olds with leukaemia, while we were being swept up into the sky in that big hot air balloon, that I could have looked toward you, past the loud congestion of warm air, and tell you just how much I would live my life for you. At Camp Quality, when we sat on the top of your bunk bed, above our volunteer companions who couldn't understand us, I wish we could again have our discussions about chemotherapy, four-syllable drug names, radiation protocols, blood products, and bone marrow transplants. I wish that I could have told you then, that one day I would walk the medical corridors once more, but this time as a professional – proficient with all the medical lingo looking after my own patients daily.

I remember the very first day we met, back in 1993. We immediately 'clicked' because we had the same diagnosis, and it was not long before we became known as the 'Troublesome Twosome', joined at the hip in every moment. We became best friends almost instantly, and you were the first friend who truly saw me for who I was, even past my bald head which was interrupting every other relationship that I was able to participate in at the time. As we soared up high in that hot air balloon, I knew that we had something special.

I wish that we could have gone on together forever, laughing at each other each camp we met, making our special memories. You were such a special friend to me, and you truly understood what I was going through. If only I could have told you, when we were teenagers and you were still smiling, just how much you always meant to me. Even though I somehow knew that I was losing you, seeing your beautiful personality through your pale and puffy chemotherapy face, somehow I still believed deep down that you would still pull through. I dreamt that we would both make five years' remission together. I continued to live in denial. Even though I was fighting my own battles as a teenager, you were still fighting bravely through every round of chemotherapy. When you did leave, it seemed so sudden, and I never had the chance to say goodbye to you.

What right did I have to stay when you couldn't? Why would God take you and not me? No matter how hard I tried, I could not understand the ruler of the heavens. The survivorship guilt that followed me after you left felt more unbearable at the time than having leukaemia to begin with. I tried to cope as best I could, but nothing seemed to help. Eventually, I turned to music, and listened repeatedly over and over again to U2's hit 'With or Without You'. I felt like I couldn't live with you, watching you go through so much pain after you relapsed, but I also felt like life would never be the same again without you. I sang and cried on the bathroom floor for weeks, so nobody else would see my suffering. Even though you were not the only one of us who didn't make it, you certainly meant the most to me.

I had been stung by the fragility of life at such a young age, but I never let go of the special memories we forged together. I fought to keep going through the pain and I pretended to pay attention in classes, even though all I could think of was life's larger lessons which didn't seem to deal fairly. I eventually did finish high school. I even put glitter in my hair to go with a lovely chap from physics to our Year 12 formal.

As a child I had walked what seemed like endless shopping malls, selling leukaemia bear badges for The Leukaemia Foundation and yellow daffodils to raise money for The Queensland Cancer Fund on Daffodil Day. Nevertheless, this still didn't seem like enough, after all that medical research had given me. Through my teens, I had spent time as a cancer advocate, speaking publicly amongst famous sports stars, coaches and other prominent members of the public – sharing my story for those like you who never had the opportunity to do so. Around the time of my high school graduation, I was selected as a Queensland Cancer Fund 'Seize the Day' Award recipient, and at 18 I went back to Camp Quality as a volunteer to mentor my own camper, a young girl who had recently lost her sister to cancer at just the age of 9. I volunteered to be featured in many newspaper articles and spoke publicly at Griffith University's research 'Thank You Day'.

I chose to live my life as if my glass were half-full, even though I saw others around me perspiring over what seemed so empty. Even though you were no longer with me, I cherished the fact that I could always remember you. If you couldn't live your life, I would live a life for you, and I vowed early on to make the most of every breath I took.

I knew that my journey had to mean something, and I went on to study Radiation Technology before becoming the youngest registered Radiation Therapist in Australia at the age of 19.

Helping other cancer patients along their own journeys seemed to also help me. I loved each one of my patients, especially learning about each of their stories. Just like you and me, not one of them deserved to have cancer, but I admired them as they kept going bravely on, struggling with the pain and side effects of treatment, but still coming again each day to complete the rest of their treatment. It was a privilege to see them smile each time I met with them, while working alongside my colleagues to help them continue through their treatment and the ungaugable uncertainty of their long-term health outcomes. Their courage gave me hope and resilience, and helped me live each day with gratitude and conviction. I knew that life could be short, and I was determined to make the most of each day I had.

If you couldn't live your life I would live a life for you, and I vowed early on to make the most of every breath I took. You know I was never much of a sportswoman. I had never been allowed to participate at school sports because I had no platelets, so I was terribly cumbersome and uncoordinated. Well, you will be surprised when I tell you that eventually, I did find a sport to participate in. I joined my local lifesaving club and volunteered to train as a lifesaver, keeping the water patrolled so others could swim with more safety. I joined with my cousins and formed a Junior Surf Boat group, and we even earned medals when we raced competitively in the Junior Surf Boat Championships.

You know I grew up on the beach, with salt water through my hair and waves that crashed heavily along the shore. It was wonderful to try to tame the water, and I even eventually bought myself a big, blue surfboard, though standing and surfing was never going to be my strong point. Nevertheless, I loved to paddle and swim amongst the dumpers and ocean swell. I lived close to the beach and bought an apartment to share with my housemate. I lived high on a hill in a street called 'Doubleview'. I liked that it had views from either side, and I enjoyed comparing this to my life experiences. At night I often looked up into the deep, dark sky off my balcony, wondering just which star you were sitting upon.

My young adulthood was a chapter of self-discovery, and I did most of this through my local community. Eventually I stopped asking the heavens why they had left me behind, and I began to change the direction of my sails, in order to transform my life into one that was more fulfilled, full of love and courage, passion and vitality. I decided to give back to my community, and I was nominated to receive my first Rotary Youth Leadership Award (RYLA), attending their leadership camp amongst the local rainforests. For three consecutive years, amongst other inspiring young leaders of my district, I was able to share experiences, hear their stories and develop life skills that would continue to serve me well into my early adulthood.

I was honoured each year that I was selected, but felt most humbled when I was nominated as the only Australian representative to travel to Gallipoli with 25 other international members to celebrate the 90th anniversary of this ANZAC battleground. To be able to make so many special friendships with those travelling with me, and to stand directly on the land on which so many of our own soldiers gave their lives so bravely, was something that I will never forget. I went on to travel solo further throughout Europe, and learnt more about each country's history, architecture and geography. I went to the castles of Switzerland and the mosques of Turkey, and experienced the amazing food and language of Germany, amongst others. Each time I have travelled, it has helped me to become the well-rounded person I am today, able to appreciate so much of the vast array of cultures that we have established in our world.

These chapters of my life were truly fast-paced and arguably packed for my young age, when I eventually decided to go back to university and study post-graduate medicine at the age of 23. I began like many others, wide-eyed, innocent and ready to scoop up information, not knowing entirely about the adventure on which I was about to embark upon. I was invigorated by the immensity of the knowledge I would eventually need to grasp, the mentors who encouraged me along my journey, and the opportunities I had to learn about people, their physiology and their medical stories that brought them to my doctor's room. I was fascinated by the working of each human body system, the influence that disease could have on this finely tuned instrument, and the impact that clinical acumen and medical therapy, combined with human compassion, could have on each and every individual passing through my care. With dedication, passion and commitment, I gradually learnt how to understand each patient's presentation, listen to their concerns, and collaboratively work with them to navigate their next best step along their medical journey.

Medical school was such an important opportunity for me, and one that I was truly appreciative of. However, despite fairly earning my position in the program, and being selected by the university singly in order to speak publicly at events and media releases, there was a part of me that felt like I wasn't ever going to be good enough. I loved being around other intelligent individuals, all enthusiastic to learn and develop professionally, however, I still felt inferior to those around me – even without evidence to support this hesitancy. Perhaps it was the immensity of the information; maybe it was the long hours I needed to work outside of university in order to pay for my accommodation. In hindsight, I feel that it was due to a complexity of factors. The truth was that, for whatever reason, after being such an independent, high-achieving individual, studying medicine was sadly the beginning of a time when I began to lose my confidence and self-esteem entirely.

The reality was that we were all travelling our own journeys, and some of my other colleagues may not have been doing well either. However, we never felt we had the courage to admit it, and we continued battling on even when it seemed hard. Soon we would be full-fledged doctors, walking the hospital corridors with general registration. In five short years we would be deemed safe and responsible to work alone clinically, taking care of people whose family members were members of our community. Medicine was certainly not easy, but what a privilege it was to have others around me to support me, putting their faith in me when they were at their most vulnerable. Each encounter with each patient was humbling, and even when it was tough it seemed worth it. I had initially set out to help others, and with integrity I continued this objective.

Having lost my confidence, you will understand my surprise when I managed to navigate the long selection process to join the Royal Australian Air Force (RAAF) medical training pathway in 2008. I had learnt about the opportunity at a local student conference, and I was one of eight chosen based on merit, leadership and potential that year, to join the program and train to eventually become an Aviation Medical Officer. As you know I have always enjoyed flying, so whether it was flying with you in a hot air balloon or flying with other servicemen and women in helicopters, C17s and F111's, I have always loved the feel of the wind in my hair up above.

In the RAAF I was trained and received exposure to experiences that I never would have dreamed of before. I wore my uniform each day with pride, as I proceeded through each part of their training program. I met my husband when I was first posted to Townsville, and I learned from others while passing mandatory courses and officer training. I spent over 10 years in the RAAF, knowing deep down that I was serving a small but important role of service to my country.

Life in medicine, in both the RAAF and the community, wasn't what I had envisioned it to be – it was so much more. Celebrating the end of our degree was like receiving a trophy for climbing the red magnificence of the Indigenous Uluru. We were so proud of our achievement, and the fact that our study seemed to now be over, even though in reality it had only just begun. Little did we know it at the time, but the upcoming journey of medicine as a career, would be more like climbing the top of Mount Everest in Nepal. With or without oxygen, the journey ahead was going to be like riding a roller coaster of emotions, both good and bad along the way.

I completed my Internship at Townsville Base Hospital, a Queensland Health facility in Far North Queensland, providing almost 600 beds to service the local and rural community. As the largest urban area north of the Sunshine Coast, I began my first rotation in general medicine, admitting patients with complex medical conditions and of varied age and background. Most patients had multiple co-morbidities and cultural diversity including Indigenous Australians and international migrants. I was 26 at the time, and while I felt prepared enough to take on the role, I had worked fewer than three short weeks when I rostered on my first overnight shift with two other interns during the night of Cyclone Yasi.

Initially, our night went well. After the few short weeks we had worked, we vaguely knew the hospital layout and had gained confidence in meeting our Registrars and Consultants for the term. We had taken bloods and placed our first cannulas and learnt how to order a multitude of pathological and imaging investigations to look after our patients. We stood tall as we walked up and down the corridors, not with arrogance, but with our new identities. It had taken years of preparation in order to get here, and we were proud of the journeys we had travelled so far. We were now responsible for each and every one of our actions, and we scrambled to keep learning every moment when we were unsure.

Despite the nerves that accompanied working through darkness, not to mention the fact that we had been rostered on during the wrath of such a huge natural disaster, I felt calmed by the company of my two colleagues. One was tall, Indigenous and kind to me, and the other I did not know well but seemed both calm and competent. We had arrived early due to the heavy rain that was already pelting down – in fact we wondered if our cars would actually remain stationary. As we sat upstairs, grateful that we were in a large strong building as we watched the cyclone gain more and more ferocity, the sheer severity of the winds made the palm trees bow down, and we were thankful that we were not home alone.

It was not long before I received an alarm from my pager. I rushed downstairs to get to the unwell patient who had abdominal pain. She was not a patient I knew, and she was unable to give me a good history due to her pain. I listened carefully to the nurse's concerns, and felt her abdomen as I ordered urgent pathology and imaging immediately. The patient had what we refer to as an 'acute abdomen' – and it was not so important for me to understand the cause, rather to order relevant investigations and to notify my Registrar that the patient was deteriorating. I later found out that she had suffered from a post-operative intra-abdominal bleed, and I was relieved that I had managed the case well even though my nerves felt like they had been getting the better of me. All those years at university studying had helped, even though it was still difficult to watch my actions being scrutinised a few weeks later when her case was presented at 'Grand Rounds'.

Medicine and life had their similarities. As Forrest Gump would have put it, 'life is like a box of chocolates – you never know what you are going to get'. Just as I never knew just which patient would line up outside my door each morning, I also never knew just which curve ball life was going to throw at me. I decided to let fate have its opportunity, and I spent the next three years working and travelling through far north Queensland and the Northern Territory. I got married at a beautiful lake in Mount Isa, and I had family and hospital staff come to watch our ceremony. We bought our first home instead of going on a honeymoon, and celebrated often, imagining what our next journey would bring.

Just 10 years later, my husband and I can look back upon this time and how truly special it was to both of us. We had achieved what we had wanted to and even more. We started a family and have two wonderful, healthy children to keep us young as we get older. We have learnt the lesson that the journey of life is truly amazing and unpredictable, but it has treasures along each side of your footpath if you are willing to stop and take hold of them. Our children teach us every day, and help to remind us of what is important.

As far as medicine is concerned, it too has its life cycle and certain predictability. I have worked in many hospitals over the years, but one of the most special moments I have been privileged to be a part of was the care of an elderly lady referred to our team for palliation, after the decision had been made to cease further transfusions and treatment for her leukaemia. She reminded me of you, as just like you and I, she too was suffering from Acute Lymphoblastic Leukaemia (ALL). She was the last patient I would treat before going on maternity leave for my second child, and she continued her battle, even though we were all aware that her bone marrow was becoming infiltrated, and she was weak from trying to keep on going. Her son and granddaughter lived locally and visited regularly, but we all knew that it would only be a matter of days before she would journey to heaven. In both assisting her family to come to terms with her palliation, and helping to adjust her drug regimen on a daily basis, I felt so humbled to be able to help her achieve comfort, and to say goodbye to those loved ones she wanted to see just one last time.

Just as for the words of *The Lion King*, it is the circle of life that continues to move us all. Sometimes very sad things happen and leave us in despair, looking for answers. Sometimes life surprises us and leads us on to more opportunities. No matter what, we can only hold onto hope; and look to the stars above when we are struggling for guidance. However, if we do not make the most of our minutes and hours, time will surely continue to pass us by.

And so, Tanya, I finish this letter to you – so grateful that you were such a special part of my childhood. I learnt so much around you and I will always see you as the strong warrior who battled against all odds to fight your leukaemia. I will always remember the times that we shared together, and the qualities of life which we endeavoured to live by. You helped me to understand that happiness is not just an emotion, but it is a journey that we all must choose to embark upon.

You will always be someone special that I cherish and remember. Love always,

Jessica

CHAPTER 6

My way

DR LAND PHAN
GENERAL PRACTITIONER

**For my mum (*'mẹ*),
who still believes in me every single day,
and who showed me that anything is possible
if you have a little bit of hope.**

"She's asking for you...please. She won't speak to anyone else."

I quickly glance at my appointment book. If I leave soon, I'll probably be able to see her during my lunch break.

It might be the last time I do.

"Okay, get the family together. I'll be there in ten."

Adrenaline starts to pump through my veins and I can feel my heart racing. I feel like I've run a marathon, even though I know it's just me overthinking. *Why me? How bad is she?*

I think back to our last consultation, when I approved her driver's licence. She had actually been quite well and we had chatted about her grandkids whilst I measured her blood pressure. She had started seeing me because I "explained things." I had met her about five years prior while her regular doctor was away, and she had kept coming back since.

I wished that one day I'd be as good as she was at eighty.

"Aren't you having lunch today?" my nurse asks as I pack my bag and grab my car keys.

"I've got a home visit – last minute, but maybe I'll grab something on the way back," I respond, making my way out. My throat feels tight, dry, and uncomfortable, but I know that I'll regret it if I don't do this.

Andrea pauses for a moment and notices my knitted brows and pursed lips.

"I'll come for a ride and we can have something together after. You might need me."

I'm grateful for her company. We didn't get along initially, with our own ways of doing things and having to adjust to each other while our roles overlapped caring for patients – but "nurse" and "doctor" are not the only terms we know each other by now. We are both mothers, daughters, advocates, and we both seek to provide the best care for our patients. I'm once again reminded of how working in the healthcare profession has brought the most dedicated, nurturing, and inspiring people into my life. I couldn't do this without my village – and I'm so glad to have found mine.

The house is reminiscent of the one in *The Castle*, a typical suburban house in varying states of decay. There is a proud Australian flag out the front.

It reminds me of my first home visit as a medical student, when my very Anglo-Saxon, very male, registrar had paused and looked at me as we both stared at the house in front of us with the very large sign at the front emblazoned with Pauline Hanson's "ONE NATION."

We'd both burst into laughter.

I hadn't known how else to respond due to the sheer absurdity of the situation. The patient had been lovely in the end as we checked the intravenous antibiotics he was having for his diabetic foot infection, but I would never forget his final parting words as he enveloped me in an enormous bear hug and bellowed (an attempt no doubt to bridge the divide of our obvious differences): *"I freakin' love fried rice!"*

I push the memory away in mirth as we make our way in, and the walls seem to close in on me as we walk down the hallway. We round the corner, and finally, we are together.

She lies in her bed, and I can see from her crumpled sheets and clothes that she hasn't left it in a while. She's lost a lot of weight. Her family is huddled outside in desperation and sadness because she's made up her mind. They miss her already.

"Do you know who I am, Nora?" I ask, tentatively holding her hand in mine.

She turns and looks at me with the same bright eyes and smiles in recognition.

"I haven't gone daft. Thank you for coming, doctor."

My nurse is already on the other side of the bed assessing the situation, her eyes taking everything in and her hands busy propping the patient up in order to check for pressure sores while helping her get into a different position.

"Let's get you into something more comfortable, shall we? Would you like some water? A cuppa?"

"Water, please."

"Nora..." Words fail me. I struggle in my inexperience. Nothing I say feels adequate. It is hard to find the words to convey what I'm trying to ask, but I try anyway.

"Would you like to stay home...are you comfortable here?" We both know what I mean.

"Yes...please," she manages to breathe out, "I would like that very much."

A vision of her frail body under fluorescent lights, rushed in on a gurney, fills my head. She is alone, confused, and frightened. Yet, I've been a doctor for almost ten years, so I find myself battling the instinct and compulsion to do something. Anything. I feel like I have to try my hardest to swim against the tide to avoid being swept away in the constant current of finding, fixing, treating.

Could we save her?

The COVID-19 pandemic has changed everything. She would likely need ICU and no one – none of her five children, nine grandchildren, and four great-grandchildren – would be able to see her. There would be endless questions, interruptions, decisions, and devices involved. There would be no peace, and time – time is already so precious right now.

We could – but does it mean we should?

I squeeze her hand one last time to find the strength to do what I must, and the family, the patient, and I all breathe a collective sigh of relief.

There are tears as we gather in the living room, and the irony of the name doesn't escape me. On paper in medical-ese, it is another *"family conference held with those who have Guardianship and Power of Attorney to discuss advance care planning."* In real life, we are just human beings trying to do the right thing for the people we care for.

While driving back to the practice, my mind is taken back to a multitude of times when I'd felt uncomfortable, out of place, and numb but had been forced to keep on going.

"You shouldn't be here," he quipped as he looked down at my abdomen, "in your condition." I was 32 weeks pregnant with my first child, attending a family friend's funeral, and hadn't even realised there were taboos in Vietnamese culture around these things, having grown up in Australia.

The thought hadn't even crossed my mind that new life and death were never to meet.

In my practice, it was quite a regular occurrence, actually. My mind had been forced from one life to the next on a daily basis since I became a medical student and started my hospital rotations. It was unspoken, but death was always around, so much so that to a degree when I look back now, I can definitely say that we simply had to learn to unsee, unfeel, and disassociate every day so that we could keep taking one step in front of the other to finish our clinics, shifts, and rotations.

It was the only way; or so I thought for a number of years.

I'm broken out of my reverie as I receive a text and my phone lights up. I glance at my phone and see the picture of my son on the screen background, smiling and bouncing with all of his two teeth. My emotions shift as I remember to breathe and smile again.

I'm so glad I found another way through – through friendships with other junior doctors and through supportive registrars who hadn't forgotten what it was like to be on the bottom rung of the ladder running the Ascites Liver Clinic alone on your first day on the job. I found that I could feel again, and that it wasn't weak to feel scared, hurt, and tired.

We all felt it, but we were together, and better for it.

At times, it felt like I was in a relationship with my team for several months: we rounded together, ate together, and the majority of my daily phone calls and messages were from them. Then I'd change rotations into a different part of the hospital and we would never speak again.

I learnt that I needed to depend on myself. I found a piece of myself I never knew existed and somehow, through the dark endless corridors and cacophony of pagers...

I found my husband.

I still remember how our gaze met in the empty lunch room, both of us trying to find a quiet place to eat and gather our thoughts before heading back out into the emergency room fray. It wouldn't be the last time we did this. The conversation felt natural and light, in contrast to the never-ending stream of suffering that awaited us outside those doors.

It was this gentle, considerate understanding of each other's needs that I still cherish to this very day.

Some things are felt, rather than said.

***

That night, I find it difficult to concentrate. I try to read after putting my son to bed, and I'm only a few pages into a book called *Patient Centered Medicine: A Human Experience*, but I can't stop thinking about the words in front of me by one Norman Cousins. I keep reading and reading them again and again. They resonate deeply with me, and I am reminded of the power that words have to connect, heal, and bring us together across time and space. I'll never meet the writer of these words, and they will never meet me, but I feel like a changed person after coming across this:

I pray that you will never allow your knowledge to get in the way of your relationship with your patients. I pray that all the technological marvels at your command will not prevent you from practising medicine out of a little black bag if you have to. I pray that when you go into a patient's room you will recognize that the main distance is not from the door to the bed, but from the patient's eyes to your own – and that this distance is best travelled when the physician bends low to the patient's fear of loneliness and pain and the overwhelming sense of mortality that comes flooding up out of the unknown, and when the physician's hand on the patient's shoulder or arm is a shelter against darkness.

I pray that, even as you attach the highest value to your science, you will never forget that it works best when it serves your humanity. For, ultimately, it is our respect for the human soul that determines the worth of our science.

This. This is who I want to be.

***

The next week she was gone.

The conversation was light, warm, and collegial with the mortuary workers. In our line of work, we did sometimes cross paths, albeit fleetingly. I signed Nora's death certificate and suddenly became overcome with emotion again.

I was confused as to what really struck me about this patient in particular when I'd lost so many others before. Although I had been affected each time, something about this time felt different.

Had I done enough?

I picked up the phone.

"John, could I have a word?"

"Of course, should I come over now?" He sounded concerned.

I rarely ever called, even though we share the same wall.

Once the barricades were down, the floods came, and a part of me felt sorry for my older male colleague as he was clearly uncomfortable. He was silent the entire time I presented my case. This was probably not the corridor consultation he expected.

I felt ashamed and weak. *Why oh why had I called him?!*

I waited for the criticism.

But it never came.

"This is what makes you a good doctor. You've done much more than I would have!"

My tears turned into a sort of choked sob-laugh and he found a quick exit, no doubt glad to be rid of me. I felt lighter and turned back to the computer, trying to steady my breathing and look as if nothing had happened for the afternoon list.

Later, I'd be very glad I had decided to be vulnerable and show my innate humanity. Little did I know, the following week, I'd be the one in his position.

***

On the day of Nora's funeral, I decided to finish my morning list a bit earlier to attend.

My first one as an actual, full-fledged GP with no "boss" to report to, independent and accountable for my own patients.

It was a strange milestone to mark, but I'd learnt to embrace the strangeness of life a long time ago and mark points on my journey as a way of remembering where I'd been: sort of like a mental trail of breadcrumbs that I suppose was to help me see how far I'd come. At times, I'd found it was easy to forget how hard you'd worked to get where you are, when you were surrounded by highly intelligent, ambitious, and accomplished people all the time.

The sky was a brilliant blue, and I could feel the heat from the sun warm on my skin when I arrived at the funeral. I felt like I was intruding on an intense, private family moment. I tried to keep my composure, but the myriad of emotions fighting for space within me began to bubble more and more, as I listened and learnt more about this woman's wonderful life. I'd only been there for the last ride, five years of what was definitely a story to remember, and it made me feel sad, embarrassed, and small to realise I'd barely scratched the surface of her. In the grand tapestry of her life, there were so many encounters and memories more worthy and important to celebrate.

I hadn't saved this woman at all. Why had she wished me to be present? How could I call myself her doctor?

Frank Sinatra's "I Did It My Way" played through the speakers, and I started to remember the person she was. It was so fitting.

My own memories of her felt so inadequate, though: because, I thought to myself, out of all the people in the room, I felt like I'd known her the least.

I hadn't known her as she'd carried her family across the world to find a better life. I didn't know the comfort of her hands apart from touching them to check her pulse or do a skin check. I didn't know her favourite songs or movies. I didn't know her as a hard worker, or remember the words she'd read to me growing up. I knew her only in past medical history, in blood pressure readings, and in specialist appointments.

Staring at her photo, it dawned on me that it wasn't about me at all: and my feelings changed to awe and humility. She had walked in and out of my life, minutes at a time, leaving an imprint on me forever. She instigated in me a realisation and new chapter and maturity in my career. It was a privilege to witness this everyday occurrence because I knew I would never look at a patient the same way again.

I suddenly realised that I *cared*. I'd just really *cared*. This simple, yet life-changing realisation took me so much by surprise that I sat in stunned silence for a moment. This understated, barely appreciated and immeasurable quality in a doctor was something that I realised I'd totally forgotten about: compassion. It just wasn't something that you can sit an examination on or top your grade in. It wasn't exactly something you can put on your resume or CV, and how do you even get better at it anyway?

To Nora, though, it hadn't mattered that I hadn't gotten perfect scores in all my examinations, or that I didn't know all the dermatological conditions that ever existed, or that I couldn't memorise *Robbins and Cotran*.

For her, it had been enough.

I was enough.

The service finished and the family were grateful but distant. I'd never met them in any of my visits with Nora in the years preceding her death, which likely said more about her fierce desire for independence rather than anything else.

It was because of Nora that I remembered my raison d'etre in becoming a doctor.

How do we adequately condense over 80 years of life onto a page?

We can't.

We must realise that we may be the ones conducting the interview to write the story, but the person living and breathing it every day: they are the ones who actually have to live it. The compartmentalisation, structure, and management is how we attempt as doctors to make sense of a lot of information. With time limitations, we pore over the patient's health documentation and medical file on the screen, but in doing so, we may miss the very essence of the person sitting in front of us if we do not pay attention.

Looking around the room full of people, I could see that this was a testament to that.

We collect data, take histories, examine, investigate, analyse, diagnose, treat, and manage. Over and over again. Thousands of times in our careers. We are so busy that sometimes we forget that if we had just listened in the first place and not cut off the patient after 10 seconds, that we might have found some answers: about the patient, yes, but perhaps about the world and even – if we are very lucky – about ourselves.

The psychological and social history of the patient is the component that we delegate to later down in the discharge summary – or sometimes omit entirely because of perceived lack of time and importance. Deemed too tedious, onerous, and/or in the "too hard basket" – the dreaded "social admission" or "acopia" are terms that strike fear in the hearts of any doctor, especially on a whirlwind surgical rotation.

This is where modern medicine could do so much better: to recognise that we may have missed something here, in our pursuit of the ultimate time-saving, energy-restoring cures and pills for health and wellbeing.

As I walked back to my car, I remained in a reflective mood.

I realised that medical school did not teach me that the parts I'd enjoy most about being a doctor had very little to do with doctoring at all.

My eyes met with my Anthea's red-rimmed ones as we drove away in silence, both lost in our thoughts.

I was right where I needed to be.

***

The longer I am in my profession, the more I realise that herein lies the strength, beauty, art, and challenge in general practice, in slow medicine. In building trust and relationships with families and communities again.

It has given me the opportunity to be present for others in their times of need: not just as they receive devastating medical diagnoses delivered by me and my fellow colleagues, but also when life simply goes awry around them and impacts on their health. Life is messy, unfair, awkward, confusing, and many times more often than not – cannot and does not need to be fixed by a doctor.

General practice is not the easy route and definitely not the specialty for everyone, but it has always been a draw for me, even if its name in Australia could never adequately portray the depth of what happens in our rooms. I've always felt it would be more appropriate to be called a family physician because my patients are not merely individuals: they are entire families. Generations. Suitable for all ages, 0–99 years.

I see family trees grow and change, bend and break. I tend to mothers and fathers, to people from all walks of life. I see my own self enriched by their stories intertwined with mine, as we grow together and apart. Sometimes I don't see people for years – and they come back changed by time: for better or for worse. It's always interesting and challenging because I am never sure what we will talk about on the day, even if I've known you my whole career.

To serve others is to know yourself and to be aware that you may not be ready to face what you see reflected in their eyes. The most important thing I've learnt in medicine is to become familiar with uncertainty and to examine why it makes you uncomfortable. As a perfectionist, I still wouldn't exactly call it my friend, but I now give it some respect and space to sit next to me as I practice. I know my patients expect the best of me, and I strive to give it – but sometimes, I can't honestly say if this treatment will get rid of the cancer for good, or if their dad will ever understand what it's like for them to live with depression.

However, I'll be there when and if they need to talk again. The stress and loneliness that affects us all at one point or another: these are the things that can be the disease, and the balm to soothe these ailments may actually be some humanity and connection. Having a safe place to seek help, to be heard and not judged, is important.

Science continues to march forward at an incredible pace, the body of information we have ever-expanding at rates no one human brain can fully comprehend. While it does so, our perspectives of past available scientific research shift and change continually, but one thing for me stays constant: my desire for human connection.

As a person whose career revolves around caring for people at their most vulnerable, I need to remind myself I must not lose sight of my own self as I continue doing meaningful work. The way that I carry out this work is clearly just as important to my patients as the work itself.

While I know I won't be winning any accolades for this quiet work, and my childhood dreams of flying around saving the world (although not misplaced) are indefinitely postponed since some tiny hands and feet have come into my life – I find myself at peace and content with my very un-glamourous, unassuming, ordinary work. The bread and butter is fulfilling, and those little moments aren't so little to the person who just needs some kindness in their day. Just as fear and anger can spread and impact those around us, I have discovered that so, too, can kindness.

As an introvert, I'd always been concerned I'd burn out due to the sheer volume of people I'd have to interact with every day. On the contrary, I've realised that my personality has actually served me for the better as a doctor in being able to shape what my days look like, already having a good grasp on my personal limitations, and fuelling my desire to know patients better, for longer and to develop more meaningful interactions over the span of our lifetimes.

The sign on the practice door changes once again to "Open."

Walking past the waiting room, I see familiar faces and love that I can now do that thing that amazed me with my GP supervisor as a student – the nod and silent, direct eye contact with the patient across the room that in a second communicates to them, *"I'm ready, I'm here for you, welcome,"* all at once.

I open up my appointment book for the afternoon and am surprised to see that my next patient has quite a familiar name.

It's Nora's daughter.

***

References: The book quoted in my story is a highly recommended read for any aspiring or current doctors at any stage in their life: Patient Centered Medicine: A Human Experience, by David Rosen and Uyen Hoang

CHAPTER 7

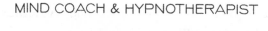

Wake up, human, it's simple

DR ANN MARIE BALKANSKI
MIND COACH & HYPNOTHERAPIST

The gentle keys being pushed in: *tap tap tap.*

My fingers move faster than my thoughts right now.

I shift my focus to the subtle rise and fall of my chest while sitting here, breathing and feeling the sensation of the keys beneath my fingertips as I type.

This brings more awareness to these words, like a sunset becoming more awe-inspiring, colorful, bright, or too beautiful for words that you are inspired to just pause and take it in.

When you gaze upon the sun setting, you enter a space with no thoughts or concerns for what you did yesterday, the day before, or even could do tomorrow.

When you focus on the simplicities of this moment, you wake up to it, just as you are reading these words and may begin to notice the spaces between the words as I point it out.

When I bring your conscious attention to the spaces or gaps of emptiness between these words, you are conscious and think about it at this very moment.

Maybe that thought causes you to pause, look, and even re-read the line above to understand what I am trying to convey by those words.

The words and spaces begin to wake you up as you notice this moment, right now, that the words you read are creating for you. As typing these words does for me, waking me up to be here with you.

I notice my lips gently quiver and curl up at the corners. Like a finger hovering over my skin, tickling those small, fine hairs. I get a lifting sensation over my body, like going over a bridge suddenly, pulling my stomach up in a sense of excitement.

Before I can even type about the image of you or simply think the thought of you, the feeling now leads me instead.

What came first, the chicken or the egg? A riddle no one knows the answer to pops in my head.

For me, at this moment, I know my feelings come before my thoughts.

My feelings and intuition have led me to this moment, now writing this to you.

Feeling takes over before my thoughts can be understood, or consciously spoken, or even typed here.

What a change it is compared to me then, which is you now.

The image of my younger self, of you, creates a sigh or sense of relief.

A lightness in my body, a wave of confidence fills my lungs like the fresh mountain air on a cool, brisk day.

My smile becomes wider as I type this, and all I can hear within myself, in a loud echoing distance, is *You did it girl, you did it, amazing you!*

A feeling radiates through my pores simply thinking of you. The only word that could describe the divineness of it all is – love.

Knowing now that all you truly needed then was love and acceptance for who you were then and are now as me.

Of all the times, my dear younger self, that you needed this guidance, it was during your adult years in peak frustration while going through medical school.

I can't recall a single human being around that knew exactly what you were going through. I highly doubt anyone could even guess.

They usually took you for the "girl next door", the one that was raised with two parents, went to church every Sunday, and maybe gathered at the dinner table with those fancy cloth napkins and fine china.

You were always well put together, with your hair nicely tucked back, light makeup around your eyes, and no lipstick, 'cause it would wear off easily.

You constantly needed to remind yourself to stand up straight and tall, even though you were slightly below the average woman's height.

On those days you wore your scrubs, even though you had your white coat on, you were still referred to as a nurse, when the men usually were called doctor.

The male domination of the field didn't bother you so much; it was more bothersome that everyone around or in your class seemed to have more confidence in themselves, or seemed to question themselves much less than you did.

Do you remember when your shoulders slouched forward, so low your chest could cave in?

You felt like one of those travel shopping bags you fold up and hide away in your car or junk drawer and forget about.

Your heart pounded so hard you could hear the whooshing of the blood passing by your ears and throat, creating a lump within it, too.

You would freeze up, unable to handle all those overwhelming thoughts in your mind, and would be extremely reactive to any emotions that came up, overthinking it.

Who could blame you, though – it was not your fault!

You are such an idiot.

You are a high school dropout and didn't even finish the 9th grade.

You had to study more than everyone else to get through undergraduate school.

How can you think you will actually be a good doctor?

Everyone is so much smarter than you.
You are a fraud.
You are not good enough.
Just hide yourself.
You are worthless.
You can't help anyone because you can't even help yourself.

I know you didn't even realize you were telling yourself these horrible things.

You would never even say such stuff to your friends, but you said these negative things to yourself every time you doubted yourself, every time you questioned yourself.

How could you not know what you did not know, and what you did not realize you were doing?

Those negative thoughts became so habitual.

Your body would clench down in anticipation of all those "what ifs" running through your mind, like that endless chasing scene of the coyote and road runner.

Your thoughts and emotions all ran away from each other, not knowing how to communicate, how to listen, or how to just understand.

What if you fail your board exams?
What if you don't get into a residency?
What if you can't be a doctor?
What if you wasted all your time and money?

Well, my dear younger self, what if it all happens? Because it will.

You will fail – multiple times at that!
You will not get into residency.
You will not be practicing as a traditional medical doctor.
And it will seem like a waste of time and money.

However, you will have to learn to trust.

Just know you are being guided and that the failures need to occur.

Those times you fall down provide the lessons you need to understand and gain the mental fortitude to stand up taller and stronger.

Without experiencing the depths of pain, hurt, or sorrow, you will not be able to comprehend the depth of love, peace, and joy.

It is all energy and emotions; if you block one, you will block all.

And, just like when you were 16, working overtime as a grocery store clerk, you could never have imagined the idea of going to college or even going to medical school.

You were too focused on simply surviving and managing expenses like rent, water, and utilities and all of those life necessities most teens don't typically need to think about: toilet paper, cleaning supplies, sanitary pads, and food.

You grew up quite quickly, and even though you will want to compare yourself to others your age, the comparison only needed to be with you.

Your journey started from a different place, and it didn't matter how many miles more you felt like you needed to go to "catch up". The thing that always mattered most was to just keep walking forward.

Follow your gut feeling, that subtle, quiet voice telling you *this is NOT you, move on.*

Like the time you experimented with drugs, used pills, got drunk more than a few times.

At 14 and with no supervision, the freedom could be overwhelming, but it also opened you up to people, places, and situations that would teach you to not judge that which you do not know truly.

Like Shawn: if anyone can be a testament to "not judging a book by its cover", he was it.

You saw Shawn's kind, soft, genuine side and his need for love and acceptance, even though he was a drug dealer.

It was quite hard for you to imagine him being a brutal person, after getting to know him, even though he looked that way, with the teardrop tattoo under his eye.

Everyone seemed to love him, or maybe it was simply respect for or fear of him because of how he looked.

But you heard something when he spoke: in his word patterns or choices, you heard insecurity and abandonment.

Shawn clearly yearned to connect with others and be accepted. For him, that was through drugs and in that community.

You had a tendency to see something good in others, but there were plenty of times you'd forget that in yourself.

Shawn had a crooked smile, and his jaw indented towards the side when he smiled.

There were visible scars and deformities all over his body, with a gaping open wound that was chronically unhealed on the outside of his leg.

There were more scars, indentations, and disfigurations on his stomach and chest.

People would gather around him as he raved about his chaotic life experiences like some gang movie; people listened intently with their mouths slightly open, mesmerized by the mere fact that he was still alive to talk about it.

Geez, this man got shot over 10 times and lived to tell these stories; he had all the scars to prove it, too.

You were mesmerized by those experiences, like being hooked into a drama reality TV series, watching those around you yell, bicker, and fight at times and party, scream, and "get crazy".

Something about it felt off, though, disconnected or fake.

The actions of those around you did not match the words said or promises made.

Hold on to these memories, because they make sense. The feeling, that sense of "offness", is you listening to your subconscious mind.

You had a sense of awareness around you. You knew what your future would be like if you kept using drugs and stayed around people like Shawn, who were simply lost.

You craved stability, a sense of structure or flow in a life that was not chaotic or messy but predictable.

Actions are predictable in people if you look, listen, and really see what it is they are telling you. Not through their words, but instead the kinds of words they choose, how they say it, and the expressions that come along with it.

These are the subconscious expressions you can sense when you walk in a room and know something bad may have happened.

This is the pattern you will pick up on with time. Just trust the feeling.

Your parents' patterns were clear for you; they were not reliable, as your mom cycled through jail or being on the streets. Your dad tried to start over, creating a new family that took up his time and attention.

You will learn to forgive and forgive, over and over again. That will be your pattern of choice. Knowing that they simply were human, un-awoken to their patterns; just as you too did not know what you did not know, they did not know either.

You did not grasp the understanding of it all, but I am here to tell you you will.

And even though you felt quite abandoned and alone at times, you kept pushing forward.

Gratitude: you become able to see the positive things in life and how the glass is half full and not half empty.

Be grateful for what you did have, instead of focusing on what you did not have... That was key!

Any hand-me-down was a blessing – clothes, kitchen supplies, or pots and pans.

Even that boyfriend of yours that you met at 15 who quit college, couldn't hold down a job, and seemed to have barely a grasp on his emotional outburst of anger. He would take it out on you by being physically aggressive, yelling, or calling you names... Yes, even he taught you to never give up.

You deserved more. You felt the call of something bigger... which is why you left when you did.

Most 18-year-olds celebrate with friends or at parties, but you celebrated your sense of freedom, alone, at home and in peace, relieved from the release of that relationship tie.

And there was that moment when you realized, because you're the one that chose to break it off, that you could create the life you live if you act and do.

Don't hold onto the guilt you may have created that makes you feel bad or like a bad person. Your intentions were always good. You are good. Be good to yourself first, and the rest will follow for you to be good for and with others.

But, most importantly, you will show others that they too are good once you realize it yourself.

You never needed to feel like a victim because you always had a choice, just like you had a choice to face your fears, decide not to be a victim any longer, and leave.

SImply follow your heart and that little voice inside telling you: *There is better... You deserve it.*

Every step you took even then taught you something and brought you closer to the reality and belief that you can do anything; you just need to want it first.

You will meet the people you need, then, to get you where you are now. Trust in that, my dear young self.

And, even though you could never imagine it then, you will continue to follow your heart and get your GED. It's quite amazing how you barely passed it after being out of school for the four years following the 9th grade.

That was the beginning, though, as you inched your way closer and closer, one day at a time

Just like you could not imagine you would ever go to college; the thought did not cross your mind, as most teens prepped for applications. You were just trying to "survive".

And now as you read this in medical school, you still survive.

You will not be able to comprehend how quickly ten years will pass. You will help people far beyond you ever thought you could. You will learn to even help yourself along the way.

You will heal from your trauma and experiences and clear your beliefs of not being good enough or feeling like a fraud.

Because you are good enough. You are authentic. And, most importantly, you are a human having a human experience, just like everyone else in this world that you have connected with. Just like Shawn, just like your mom, just like your dad, just like your ex-boyfriend, and just like you are as you read this.

Your human experience is unique to you, so you will feel alone – but you were never alone.

You always had me. Your highest self in you. Speaking to you every time you doubted and lost your sense of self. Bringing you back, waking you back up, and pushing you along the way.

I was guiding you.

I am that image of yourself that you had glimpses of, that future sense of self you created in your mind.

However, I do have to tell you, my dear young self... I superseded your image.

I superseded the expectations you had then because of the limitations you had within yourself. Only time will release those limitations.

And, just like you imagined me, your future sense of self, I now have a new image of my higher self.

My image is not what you would have expected, though.

As my dear young self, you are very limited in your views.

You are limited by the sensations you experience because you have blocked so much already.

Your experiences created certain filters over your eyes or the lens you see life through or that you see your reality as.

So if I told you that you have a book – sure, you will know you have a book, maybe because you are holding and touching it with your hands. You can feel the pages and you can see it, too. That is real to you, and therefore your understanding of reality is confirmed by this experience through these sensations.

But let's pretend that you closed your eyes, so you do not have sight, and you couldn't use your hands, so you do not have touch, and I now told you that you have a book in front of you.

You can only believe that what I am telling you is true.

But in order to do this, you first need to trust – trust in that intuitive knowingness, deep in your gut, that I am telling the truth.

A sensation, a feeling, a knowing – it is energy flowing through you and communicating many more things going on around you.

It's that energy that gives you goosebumps when you think of someone and they all of a sudden call you.

Or when you decided to not do something, for clear logical reasoning, but it turns into the best thing you could do, because it saved you from something or meant you were at the right place at the right time to meet someone that will change your life in so many ways.

So, like closing your eyes and going inward, you will learn to experience a different reality that you can not see or tangibly experience but that is nonetheless real. You only need to trust the process in knowing so.

You will feel it stronger and stronger within you, a place of connectedness.

You are drawn to it in nature because nature has this energetic connection, too.

You may shy away from the idea and find it "woo", but spirit is energy. You'll trust in it because you will experience it.

Like your heart, it radiates from your body – like when they check an EKG and can see the pulses, even when the reader is only touching your skin. Those impulses, those waves, have an electric charge, have spirit within it, and it flows out, around and in you.

Everything has spirit.

Life is an energetic force, constantly flowing in a perfect pattern of existence. You can choose to flow with it or to resist – until you finally let go and trust that you will be protected and guided even more.

It's like the leaf from a tree that holds on and may fear the idea of letting go, simply because the tree itself is all it knows. Once that leaf lets go, it glides, supported by the wind, the air, and it will gently glide to the ground.

The leaf will then be lifted and carried to new places or destinations, until there comes a day that the leaf will settle, allowing for the transformation to occur for it to be a part of earth. A part of the ground, giving nutrients and life to the soil, creating compost that feeds the flowers and trees that create the air that we breathe.

The soil gives that very nutrients to the fruits and vegetables that feed the animals or us humans.

So, you see, my young self, we are all connected. Life is connected. So, the image of what I now consider my higher self is no image; it is that very essence of existence in life. Light and love.

My dear young self, I leave you with the one simple answer within it all, within every experience, every struggle, every challenge, everything you have endured to get to this point and what you needed every step of the way.

Trust, to let go, to let be, and to let love come in.

Love is life.

So wake up, human, to the love and life you live now.

CHAPTER 8

Sawubona udokotela

DR MELANIE UNDERWOOD
EMERGENCY PHYSICIAN

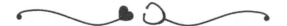

I shift uncomfortably on the hard wooden bench. I look at my watch. I've been waiting two hours.

I collapse back against the wall, close my eyes, and inhale deeply. The room is silent except for the slow, rhythmic ticking of a clock. I'm alone in this small building. The "arrivals lounge" at Matsapha Airport in Manzini, Swaziland. There is a single check-in desk, which is now deserted, and a rudimentary carousel that held the luggage of ten or so passengers who'd traveled from Johannesburg. This tiny country is nestled in the northeast corner of South Africa, sharing a border with Mozambique. Swaziland, with a population of only one million people, is one of the few countries in the world still ruled by an absolute monarchy.

A driver from the Good Shepherd Hospital has been charged with collecting me from the airport, but it's now been two hours since I landed in that old, tiny, fixed-wing aircraft. Thanks to flight delays and cancellations, I have been awake for 27 hours straight. I'm starting to appreciate that I am going to have to adjust my expectations to "African time." Things move more slowly here. I inhale again, trying to discourage the stinging tears welling up in my eyes. I don't know what to do. I don't have a phone. I don't know who to call.

How on earth did I end up here?

I know exactly how I ended up here – I'm escaping. Turning 30 this year should have brought happiness, anticipation, and excitement. It's 2008 and I've been a doctor in Australia for five years. My career is tracking nicely. I'm training to become an emergency physician and I'm good at working under pressure. I thrive on the variety, my skills are extensive and, at times, life saving. A successful resuscitation is exhilarating, even if somewhat subdued compared to the drama I passionately watched through eight seasons of *ER*. However, unlike the tv show, there is no Dr John Carter. In fact, there has not been a man in my life since I started medical school nine years ago. I have been focused on my career. Driven. Determined. However, this has all been complicated with feelings of inadequacy, of not being good enough and feeling like I just don't measure up to my peers. Perhaps that's why there hasn't been any romance in my life.

Boys don't make passes at girls who wear glasses.

Thirty isn't old, but it's the fear of never finding someone that makes my ovaries ache. I thought by now I'd have had at least some expression of interest. Perhaps it's my pock-marked skin. The brutal remains of terrible steroid-induced acne in my late adolescence. Perhaps it's my Catholic girl school education, compounded by being raised by a single mother? I simply don't know how to interact with men.

Perhaps I'm just meant to be alone. Perhaps I am not enough.

This resignation had led me to accept an offer from my best friend. A tall, dark and handsome doctor, he'd been my John Carter. Unfortunately, he also appreciated tall, dark, handsome men. Nevertheless, our friendship flourished and over lunch one day he asked me if I would consider having a baby with him. My best friend hadn't met Mr Right. He desperately wanted children – he thought I was perfect maternal material. We'd live together and raise the baby. He suggested that before we embarked on this plan, we'd take six months to go and volunteer in an African hospital together. He knew somewhere, in Swaziland. If we could survive six months together working in a foreign country, we could survive all the challenges of raising a child in an unconventional home.

I was giddy with excitement. This wasn't the arrangement I had grown up dreaming about, but it was the best I had ever been offered. I was going to have that deeply desired baby and I was going to do it with my best friend. A man who was smart, compassionate and had dreams and aspirations similar to my own. We were off to Africa and I was invigorated with hope and happiness.

Then everything imploded.

He fell in love with a man who didn't share the same dreams. We weren't going to Africa and I was left gasping with the despair that I wasn't even good enough for a gay man.

Emerging from the pain and disappointment, I decided to continue alone with the plan to work in Swaziland. Perhaps the universe was showing me its grand purpose. Swaziland had the unenviable position of having one of the highest rates of HIV infection in the world. Over 40% of the population had the virus and the average life expectancy was 40 years. If I wasn't going to partner and have babies, then I was going to fight the good fight in Swaziland.

Sawubona udokotela – hello doctor?

Disrupted from my reverie, I hear a gentle voice, in broken English, call out for me. I look up and a sheepish looking man identifies himself as Promise. He's taking me to the Good Shepherd Hospital.

I heave my suitcase into the minivan and we share our short trip along ragged roads with meandering cattle and goats. I can see impeccably dressed women walking proudly with baskets of produce perched adroitly on their heads, babies snuggly attached to their backs in cotton slings. Children chase dogs or scurry for a makeshift soccer ball consisting of rubbish tightly banded together to form a ball. I see odd little huts emblazoned with signs advertising Coca Cola or mobile phone credit. A rather confusing sight amongst the rondavels consisting of mud, sticks, and thatched roofs. I hold my breath and brace with fear as we dodge combi vans overstuffed with people haphazardly criss-crossing the roads. I smile at the irony of billboards advertising "Trust" condoms and I can't help but be perplexed by the disproportionate number of places advertising coffins and funeral services.

Within an hour, we arrive at the Good Shepherd Hospital, a collection of white-washed buildings nestled in the shadows of giant jacaranda trees. Promise escorts me to a tiny room on the hospital grounds. I savour the warmth and rejuvenation of a shower. Shortly, there is a knock at the door. Embarrassed to be wearing my Winnie the Pooh pyjamas, the director of the hospital, Dr P, who is a warm, engaging Eritrean, kisses my hands as he welcomes me to Good Shepherd. He tells me how delighted they all are that I have arrived. The doctor who oversees the medical care of all the patients is going away for a six-week holiday and I will be replacing him. My eyes widen with incredulity and a slight anxiety gnaws the base of my stomach. He looks around and tells me that I should close all the windows. "Snakes," he says with a smile. "We call this area Snake Hill." It is home to the deadly mamba, puff adders, and the occasional cobra. He bids me goodnight with another generous round of kisses to my hands and I crash in a heap on my bed, wondering where exactly I have landed.

I wake early the next morning, eager with anticipation of what lies ahead. First impressions are important and I want to appear polished despite the intense anxiety and uncertainty I feel. I almost deplete the hospital's electricity supply as I meticulously straighten my hair.

Walking towards the hospital, I notice the expanding number of patients arriving at the hospital outpatient clinic. They come in the back of trucks and utility vehicles, their limp bodies carried in by relatives or members of their village. Some are pushed in wheelbarrows. There is no ambulance service in Swaziland and this is the only means of carrying an invalid to reach medical help. I make my way through a large crowd, aware of inquisitive stares from onlookers. My white skin and long, dark hair make me an obvious mlungu (white person), my white coat and stethoscope the only clues that I'm a udokotela (doctor).

I meet the doctor I will be replacing. Dr K is a quiet, discerning man with a warm smile. A group of nursing staff jostle for a close position, as they are eager to meet the new doctor. The nurses are young, immaculate in their pristine white, meticulously starched uniforms. Their nursing caps are reminiscent of a bygone era. I soon recognise that they will be my key allies, able to translate in clinical consultations and explain cultural nuances that help me understand a country so foreign to my own.

The ward round is interminable. Bodies languishing in beds, on mattresses placed between beds and haphazardly placed in the hospital administration area. The hospital is currently over-capacity. Patients are being turned away at the doors and families are made to take their loved ones home to die. I'm recording my patient encounters to submit to my training college back in Australia. At the end of a five-hour ward round, I'm able to deduce that 90% of patients have HIV/AIDS. Their disease is complicated by tuberculosis, meningitis, and horrendous malignancies that simply aren't treatable in this impoverished nation.

How on earth am I going to be able to deal with these problems?

I'm horrified by the absence of simple medical equipment. Emesis bowls don't exist, so patients are forced to vomit on the floor, in their beds, or simply over themselves. There is a scarcity of bins for the disposal of medical sharps such as needles and scalpels. I note the cardboard box in the nurses' station that is used to dispose of used needles harbouring infectious particles of HIV. Latex gloves are difficult to access and only used in theatre.

One of the first procedures that I perform that day is a lumbar puncture to investigate a patient for meningitis. The procedure involves taking a sample of fluid that bathes the brain and spinal cord. It is usually performed under the strictest of sterile techniques. Here on the ward, there are no sterile drapes and no local anaesthetics to improve the tolerability of the procedure. I'm handed a single cotton wool ball soaked in iodine. It barely removes the dirt caked on the skin, let alone any of the microbes that colonise the surface. I have a simple spinal needle and a collection jar. The only saving grace is that the procedure is technically simple. HIV wasting syndrome has rendered the patient emaciated and the bony prominences of the spinal vertebrae are easily visualised. I am taken aback by the stoicism of the patient. She does not flinch during the procedure. My heart sinks as the turbid fluid that flows freely from the needle confirms my suspicions of meningitis. I console myself with the realisation that at least I have a diagnosis and I can treat with intravenous antibiotics.

However, not even antibiotics can save some patients. Next is a 13 year old girl who has presented with septic shock. Her well-meaning parents have taken her to one of the traditional healers and part of her treatment involved cutting the skin to release the "poison" coursing through her veins. The dirty razor blade has left her with infected wounds. Despite aggressive antibiotic management and wound care, I cannot save her. She lapses into a coma and dies shortly afterwards. The hopelessness is starting to envelope me, and my chest tightens as I watch her small body being covered in a shroud.

Another of my patients is a 33 year old woman who is bed-bound with paraplegia. Many years ago, an obstructed labour had required her to have a spinal anaesthetic for an emergency c-section. Unfortunately the procedure was complicated by infection and she was permanently paralysed from the waist down. Now she's in the terminal phase of AIDS and has profuse, watery diarrhoea. The deep pressure sores on her buttocks, the result of years of immobilisation, have now become infected with the excrement. Patients in the hospital are issued with one incontinence pad per day, but this is inadequate in the face of this horrendous diarrhoea. The woman languishes in a foul stench that permeates the ward as she slowly endures a painful, lonely death.

An 18 year old girl has presented with AIDS complicated by PCP pneumonia, a common infection seen in patients devoid of an immune system. She's doing well on her antibiotics until she develops a nose bleed. Her platelets, the cells involved in blood clotting, are critically low and she is left to bleed to death. There are no platelet transfusions available and no equipment to stop the bleeding. Bile starts to rise up in the back of my throat as I seethe with anger. The inequality and injustice of the situation are starting to paralyse me.

I return to my room at night exhausted and despairing.

I'm out of my depth.

I am managing conditions I've never seen before. With Dr K now on holidays, I am only left with my surgical and obstetric colleagues for advice. They are so overburdened and overwhelmed that their medical opinion is often rudimentary. As the only "physician" in the hospital, I am asked to consult on post-surgical, obstetric, and psychiatric patients with intercurrent HIV complications.

Every morning, I wake up tangled in sheets and dishevelled. The night terrors leave me with a haunted appearance. What is most surprising is my inability to cry. I am a renowned crier, a characteristic often seen as a weakness amongst my medical colleagues. However, here, in the face of the most horrendous humanitarian crisis, I am unable to shed a tear. Not only am I questioning my ability as a doctor, I'm now questioning my ability to feel like a normal human being.

Weeks of gruelling ward rounds and never ending outpatient clinics pass by. I'm starting to recognise disease patterns and having some success in treating conditions I have only ever read about in textbooks. The nurses find me endearing and with the implementation of some of my new ideas and morning tutorials, we are starting to become a formidable clinical team. There are moments of levity on the ward rounds. Gospel songs project from loudspeakers to accompany lunch. Nurses sing songs of praise whilst they work. One of the nurses is disappointed when she comes to my room one night asking that I become her prayer partner. I decline her request, stating that I would not be a good choice. I dare not voice my truth that, having borne witness to a disease that has decimated almost half a nation, God has ceased to exist in my mind. I smile when I see one of the surgeons walk around the hospital with his red baseball cap emblazoned with "I love Jesus." I bite my tongue and busy myself when preachers come to the ward every day with their evangelical proclamations that if the patients just turned to God, their suffering would end.

In the midst of all this, there are still moments of gut-wrenching despair. It's late one afternoon when a nurse rushes up to the weekly doctors' meeting and implores me to review a patient. It's a 40 year old woman who is a very well respected member of the local community. Her husband died of AIDS 12 months earlier and she had been left widowed with three teenage daughters. She is a devoted housekeeper for the local ophthalmologist. Initially, the woman responded well to her treatment for PCP pneumonia, but now she has developed severe respiratory distress. I race to the ward to discover the patient on oxygen but in extremis. There is little I can do as I watch her gasp her last breaths. She dies in front of me. The fifth patient we've lost that day. The woman's daughters are outside and once they hear the news that their mother has died, they are devastated. They fall to the floor, wailing. Their bodies are convulsing with grief. News spreads quickly and there is soon a mass of people all wailing, crying, and desperately seeking answers I cannot give them.

This woman's death, among so many I have witnessed here, seems to break something inside of me. A million questions race through my mind. I am traumatised, gripped with inadequacy and hopelessness. My chest heaves and bile rises to the back of my throat. If I don't escape now, I'm going to vomit and collapse with the same despair experienced by these orphaned girls. I cannot publicly reveal my weakness. I race to my tiny room. It's oppressively hot and claustrophobic. The walls are closing in on me. I tumble onto the bed, howling with a guttural anguish and helplessness.

My breakdown is cathartic, and it's a welcome relief to finally acknowledge the trauma I have been witnessing. The ravages of disease and poverty. The hopelessness of an epidemic fuelled by poor resources, cultural traditions, and misinformation. I've seen so many young girls who have been raped as a result of the belief that sex with a virgin will cure men of HIV. The South African president has claimed that showering after intercourse is a way of preventing infection with HIV. It's all confusing, frustrating, and totally out of my control.

I'm halfway through my time in Swaziland and I'm starting to not recognise myself. My compassion and empathy are starting to erode. The stigma and associated denial around HIV are infuriating. On one particularly arduous ward round, I inexplicably raise my voice in anger as one of my young patients refuses to acknowledge her newly diagnosed HIV. I implore her to accept the diagnosis and commence treatment. In a moment of desperation I tell her to look around and see that everyone else around her has HIV and she needs to fight to survive. I am ashamed of my behaviour. This is not the doctor I used to be. Whilst I may still sit on beds, hold hands and comfort the dying, I am not someone who yells and gets angry at patients. I am not that doctor. I am not that person. The cracks are starting to show. Later, out of sight of the patients, I slump into a chair and hold my head in my hands as I ask in exasperation, "Is there anything in Swaziland that is easy?"

One of my young, enthusiastic nurses ruefully replies, "It's easy to catch HIV in Swaziland."

As well as forging strong bonds with my medical colleagues and developing an affectionate admiration of Swazis, I have made strong, meaningful friendships with a number of expatriates here in Swaziland. Two passionate nurses from the USA, a medical student from Scotland, and another from Germany. An extraordinary couple from America working for the Peace Corp. They sustain me, encourage and uplift me. We become a family when family is so far away from home. In an attempt to escape the rigours of hospital life, we decide to attend the annual Reed Dance in the country's capital. A celebration of virgin girls who assemble costumes and jewellery from reeds and dance in front of the King. It's a particularly special event this year as it coincides with Swaziland's 40 years of independence from England. The King is also turning 40. He's purchased 40 new Mercedes Benz to transport officials to the ceremony. One of these officials includes his close friend, Robert Mugabe of Zimbabwe. The King is also taking a new wife. His 13th to date. He's commissioned a private jet to take his other wives, their children, nannies and bodyguards to Dubai so that they can holiday whilst he becomes acquainted with his new wife. The idea of attending the Reed Dance and, by association, condoning the event, conflicts me. Whilst a fascinating insight into Swazi culture, the event leaves an indelible picture of the chasm between all that is celebrated in the country and what is actually experienced in the day-to-day existence of Swazis. I return home from the event with an enormous headache and proceed to spend the rest of the evening vomiting.

The daily machinations of life at the Good Shepherd Hospital are starting to develop a familiarity and my confidence is building. However, I'm again rocked with uncertainty when one of the nurses from the female ward comes to see me during a particularly gruelling outpatients clinic. She informs me that one of our pregnant patients has died from her meningitis. She then proceeds to tell me that the relatives are asking what am I going to do with the unborn baby. I look up with some incredulity and ask, "Didn't you tell the relatives that the baby has also died? A baby cannot be alive in a dead mother."

She shifts uncomfortably. I can see that she hasn't told the family, but there is something else going on. I gently probe her thoughts further, only to be informed that in Swazi culture, mothers are not to be buried with their unborn children. In one horrifying moment of clarity I ask, "Am I expected to remove the baby?" The nurse looks at me, clearly understanding that this is not something I would be comfortable doing. She quietly tells me that the mortician can be asked to do it if I'd prefer. I nod my head with a silent instruction and the nurse returns to let the family know.

One of the highlights of being one of the few mlungos in town is that I am often the recipient of generous kindness and respect. When I have walked the kilometre into town to buy water and groceries, local women have sometimes offered to carry my bags and we chat together in broken English as we go. Children delight me with their innocent smiles and inquisitive requests to touch my skin and hair. I have to admit, I have blushed when young men have called me pretty or told me that they like my bum. I certainly never garnered this much attention back home. I always carry my Mary Poppins style umbrella when I walk, not in case of the rare downpour but rather as an effective weapon against local dogs and snakes. I've never felt unsafe walking into town until the day I am grabbed by a young man as I pass the local petrol station. I am paralysed with terror; he has me by the arm and is pulling me into a building. Adrenaline is coursing through my veins and I can't exhale in order to scream. Within seconds I realise that my virginity is at risk of being taken by a rapist and possibly a rapist with HIV. An explosion of rage and fear enables me to swing that umbrella and start screaming for help. I twist and contort my body and the man finally releases his grip. He smiles sardonically at me as I stumble away, the mocking smile on his face seared into my brain. He scared me, but he took nothing from me. My heart is pumping in my chest and my legs feel like they are made of jelly, but I manage to start running. I run all the way back to Good Shepherd and lock myself in my room. Lying and trembling in my bed, I stare at the ceiling for hours. Tempering my thoughts of what could have been.

It's my 31st birthday.

***

A few months have passed and I'm now back in Johannesburg Airport. I shift uncomfortably in my seat. I look at my watch. The plane returning to Australia is delayed. Reflecting on the past six months, I look around me. I'm surrounded by hundreds of people and yet still feel so alone. This all feels so surreal and I consider if I will ever be able to return to my normal life after Swaziland. I have changed. This experience has left an indelible mark on my soul. The beauty, innocence and generosity of the Swazi people have become part of me. I came to Swaziland conflicted. My identity was defined by my single status, the fear that I would never be afforded the opportunity to have children and my desire to compensate for all of that by packing my bags and using my medical skills to help save an AIDS-ravaged nation. I clearly never succeeded.

Oh, how naive I was six months ago.

The only gift I will receive today is a good dose of perspective. If there is a lesson to be learnt from all of this, it's that I am no longer defined by my marital status, my parental status, or my career status. I'm defined by my courage. My ability to persevere in the face of enormous challenges. My identity is formed by my tenacity and resilience. I can still allow myself to cry in the most tragic of circumstances, because this is what makes me human, a perceived weakness to some and yet something that sets me apart as being a truly compassionate, feeling, empathic doctor.

Boys may not make passes at girls that wear glasses, but nevertheless, I am more than enough.

CHAPTER 9

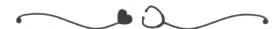

DR ERKEDA DEROUEN
FAMILY MEDICINE PHYSICIAN

Hey girl,

I know you! You're the lively, young, enthusiastic science nerd who has dreamt of being a doctor practically your entire life. You likely played with doctor kits as a wee toddler and corrected those who called it a nursing kit, stating, "No, I'm a doctor!" You probably joined extra-curricular groups geared towards students who were interested in medicine. You mapped out a plan and then worked it! I know your story because it mirrors mine. Like I once was, I know that you are excited to embark upon the journey of starting your medical career. Oh, and that you're Black.

Let me tell you a little bit about my story...

My name is Erkeda, but those that know me well call me Keda. I worked to fulfil my grandfather's dream of starting medical school, something that he mentioned with pride, as he was also accepted into medical school but could not attend due to life circumstances. I, too, yearned to serve individuals through the field of medicine. So I performed well in school and eventually transitioned to school in Boston, Massachusetts, one of the hot spots of medical education and innovation. Boy, was I excited!

If you're not familiar with Boston, it is a beautiful, historic place. Some buildings are as old as the Boston Tea Party. While the climate was cold, and it seemed as though winter lingered for nine months out of the year, there was tons to do in the city, ranging from Red Sox games to elaborate museums, to dining at phenomenal ethnic restaurants.

I was initially introduced when I moved there in a "Real World TV show-esque" way. I was chosen along with 15 strangers to live in a brownstone together, study, and avoid drama while participating in a medical school pathway program. There were many adventures that awaited me as I explored the city with my cohort, in between studying, and I was naive to think that I was ready. Those next four years would change me forever.

I share this love note with you to allow you to learn from my experience.

A Whole New World

Girl, look at you! You've worked so hard to get to this point, and now you're here. If you're like me, you may be in for a cultural awakening. I hailed from the suburbs of DC and Prince George's County, Maryland, where the community was 99% Black. To be fair, there were a total of three White people in my graduating high school class (yes, three). I could name them, but I won't in this text. My college was an HBCU (historically Black college or university), the illustrious Hampton University. I spent most of my life immersed in Black culture, in which I was the majority.

For most, medical school is an entirely different story. Well, there are four historically Black medical colleges in the US, and many of the other schools are not very diverse. In the US, Black people compose 5% of physicians, with around 3% of them Black women and 2% Black men. This number has not changed much, if at all, since 1978. My school was a little more diverse, with a little over 16 out of 200 or so of those entering the first year class being Black, including three Black students who did not enter via the special program. Medical schools are notorious for causing issues with support for Black students. We are more likely to be dismissed or expelled from school. My institution was no different. Out of the 13 of us that matriculated via that program, three of us graduated "on time."

Being "different" was a new concept to me. When they told me that Boston was one of the most racist cities in the North,

I chuckled. I didn't believe them. It did seem a little odd when I told my mentor that I had chosen to move into an apartment in South Boston, and she informed me that they had just started to allow Black people to live there in the 90s. Not the 1890s, but the 1990s. I was a sheltered Black American suburban princess. While I sought to explore diversity in this new city, I had not really had much exposure to other cultures, as I was from Prince George's County, Maryland, which has the most wealthy African Americans per capita in the US and hadI attended an illustrious historically Black college (HBCU), Hampton University. I was in for a culture shock but excited to learn about new people and that glorious new place known as "the Bean."

Racism. It's an ugly word that most want to "unsee." One may choose to look away when it does not affect them. I could not choose to do that, as a Black woman in Boston, because it was targeted towards me, both aggressively and passive-aggressively.

I entered the endeavor with a built-in support system, which is your beloved EMSSP community. I love my friends and I am fiercely loyal, but I wanted to spread my wings and get to know all of my classmates. I certainly met some amazing friends outside of my bubble, but these years would introduce me to some of the most isolating moments of my life.

You'll be met with resistance. I was...

There were feelings of isolation. Whispers and rumblings of rumors that other people could have had my spot, if it weren't for affirmative action. Even a prominent school official would write an article about minority students bringing down the scores of the students, which would later be retracted. It could have broken me, but it didn't. These experiences will shape me into who I am, allowing me to find my voice and shine my light.

Don't Dim Your Light

There will be times in which you will want to cower. Don't!

There is no better example of this than when I entered the clinical years of my training. There were some instances like when I was called other Black student's names even though we did not resemble one another in the least. There were other students that refused to join my study groups. No slights were as blatant as when I took my internal medicine rotation.

There was an instructor that was a douche. He made "pimping" a thing. Pimping is a term used in medicine when a senior medical person asks multiple different questions during rounds in order to assess a "lower level" learner's knowledge base, sometimes through public humiliation. His misogynistic tone towards me was apparent. One time after he asked me a question, in which I answered absolutely perfectly because I knew my material, he responded, "It's hard to listen to what you have to say because with a voice like yours, one would presume that you were an 'airhead', but you really understand the material." I wanted to fade into a wall because this was stated in front of a group of peers and teammates during rounds. When it was time for feedback towards the end of the rotation, he asked me what I was planning to do with my career. I told him that I wanted to work in academics. His response was gut-wrenching. He told me, "Create a Plan B because you're a) a woman and b) a minority, so it will be hard for you." Uh, YEAH, with people like him leading medicine, it would be. Therefore, I'm not going to sugar coat it. It will be hard for you, too, my dear.

Although I did not stand up for myself during that experience in my third year, I learned to never take any crap from anyone again, no matter who they were. People will try to use their positions of power against you each and every day, but you have a choice of whether or not to accept it. After sharing my experience with a mentor of mine in the medical school, the sweetest female attending physician, who also happened to be Caucasian, encouraged me to use my voice and find my power and my people. I would from then on out.

You'll Fall Down

Medical school will be one of the hardest things that you will ever do. You've likely come from the top of your class. News alert: all of your classmates have, too! Learning the volume of information from medical school work is often described as trying to drink from a fire hose. Honestly, I could not think of a better analogy. When I started my first year, I would like to say that I was thoroughly prepared. Honestly, I was not.

I was academically gifted for as long as I can remember. I didn't have to try hard to perform well in school. I mentioned earlier that I had matriculated to medical school through an early admissions program. Which meant that I had spent my entire senior year of college taking medical school-level courses prior to my "official" first year. Those classes were a rude awakening for the magnitude of studying I would need to embark upon. While I was aware that there would be academic challenges with the extent of medical coursework, I didn't account for the realities of life.

Life happens for everyone. I was no different. Aside from adjusting to the academic rigors of school, my friend and study partner became ill. It was the C word; cancer. She was diagnosed in the spring of our first year. While it was hard to wrap my mind around a young woman struggling to stay alive when she was only in her early 20s with her entire life ahead of her, I struggled to be supportive while continuing to study.

The biggest wrench in my first year came not from my friend's illness but from a family loss. My grandfather, who inspired me to enter medicine, passed away during the week of a large test. Because I was overly communicative about my stress levels, my family chose to tell me about his passing after my exam. I. Was. Devastated. I also could not fly to the funeral due to expensive flight costs and schedule coordination. Through it all, I did not ask for help. Unfortunately, my grades reflected that.

It was a caring mentor who checked on me weekly who recommended that I "get it together." As someone that was still prideful about needing help, I didn't utilize tutors as other classmates did because, for some reason it made me feel less intelligent. In actuality, it was the opposite. I definitely knew my information. I could teach the concepts to those who were acing the tests. I just didn't perform well under pressure myself. It wasn't until I hit rock bottom after failing the most important test of my life at the time, the infamous USMLE Step One test – by two freaking points – that I acknowledged I needed to reach out to someone to help myself. I finally took the advice and got a test-taking strategy consultant and figured out that my style of studying was completely wrong. I thrived in test taking after that.

You'll Find Your People

It will help to find a support system. A personal board of directors (BOD), if you will. This is a team of unofficial people who have your back. It may be your mother, a classmate, an instructor, a friend from home, a member of your church, a student a few years ahead of you in your studies. Actually, it should be a variety of individuals who have your best interests at heart, you can run ideas problems by and brainstorm with.

Like I've mentioned before, pride can sometimes get the best of you. I was not always forthcoming when I needed help. Don't be ashamed to ask for help. You are doing new and difficult things. If it were meant to be simple and easy, you would not need to do it.

My personal BOD was a smorgasbord of great folks. Of course, I started my medical school journey with familial support and the aforementioned EMSSP group, but I also met a ton of wonderful classmates and even folks in the community outside of school. One of my greatest findings was my beloved Student National Medical Association (SNMA).

The SNMA was founded in the 1960s, when Black students were not allowed to join the American Medical Student Association (AMSA). They are committed to supporting current and future underrepresented minority medical students, addressing the needs of underserved communities, and increasing the number of clinically excellent, culturally competent, and socially conscious physicians. Its focus gave me a voice, a support system, and a way to live out my purpose of serving the community. I served in many roles on local, regional, and national levels. Outside of the mission, it also gave me a group of students who became friends who were dealing with the same things.

I found my way. By the end of my time in medical school, I matched into my number one choice for residency in Family Medicine. I was awarded several scholarships, but one that I hold most dear is the Humanism in Medicine Award. All of the struggle wasn't in vain.

You'll Reach Back

Experiencing the aforementioned obstacles changed me tremendously. I evolved from a shy, quiet student into a fierce advocate for those who could not advocate for themselves. For example, a very high-level doctor in the medical school wrote an article blaming Black students for the drop in their school entrance testing stats, something that was not true, as many of the students weren't required to take the exam for entrance into the medical school. I learned to take these aggressions and thrive in spite of them. Now, I mentor medical students to help overcome their obstacles. As much as things change, a lot of things remain the same. There are tons of students who continue to experience some of the same things that my Black classmates and myself went through.

Not only did I learn to advocate for medical students, I truly decided to advocate for my patients. I became a Family Medicine physician, one who is indeed known as a "jack of all trades." What is not mentioned about the specialty is that primary care is one of the most intimate jobs that there are. I have been present in some of the most private moments of a person's life: when a new life is born, as a new diagnosis of cancer is made, when someone finds out that they beat their diabetes goals, when another takes their last breath. I've been there during times when patients reveal that they cannot afford medications or food. Finding my voice allowed me to work to find a voice to help others. You too will have a chance to help your patients, perhaps in a different manner than I.

My experiences caused me to take my advocacy outside of the clinical room and into the boardroom. When my colleagues were struggling to gain proper support in the workplace, I helped lead a successful unionization effort. I transitioned out of a traditional medicine space to find my people once more in the field of tech against some naysayers. Now, I am able to use my voice to help impact the voiceless from a perspective different than one from clinical interactions. I've turned my trials into testimonies in order to empower others to believe in themselves and conquer their dreams.

Your story was meant to uplift others. I cannot wait to witness the things that you will do.

Love,

Erkeda

CHAPTER 10

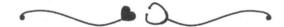

I remember

DR FAYE JORDAN
EMERGENCY PHYSICIAN

As I arrive in the Children's Emergency Department, I casually wander through the waiting room to gauge the start of my day. I breathe easy, relaxing into an effortless walk to the handover room, my spirits lifted by the fairy-tale characters that adorn the walls. Today will be a good day. Just a couple of families waiting to be seen. A quick glance reassures me that no one is seriously unwell. We settle into our familiar banter as we pull up the triage and tracking screen on the computer. My night staff are spent and keen to get away to the comfort of their beds, despite the daylight hours ahead.

A new triage pops onto our screen. A category 2. The triage nurse must be concerned. As I read, a sense of dread pervades the pit of my stomach. A precious little one, only a few months old, unexplained bruises, a swollen leg, and pale. This child has caused disquiet amongst the nurses. They, too, can sense something is wrong.

The baby is the colour of the hospital wall. His mum and dad cradle him in their arms, pleading their eyes pleading with me to tell them everything is alright. My heart sinks, my throat tightens, and my mouth becomes dry. Please, no. Not today. I don't want to tell another family their precious little one has just stepped off a precipice onto the roadway to premature death. A day that will be etched into their memory forever. A day that somehow will become woven into the tapestry of their life, not as Christmas Eve, but as the day they went to the Children's Emergency. The day everything changed. No. Not today. I will not accept this news today.

Today will always be remembered as the day they were told that their child had cancer. Along with every Christmas Eve, for all their tomorrows. Today will be the very worst day of their lives. Worse still, this will be the beginning of a hideous journey, day one on a journey of endless needles, drugs, torturous procedures, and unwanted side effects. Of gazing into their beautiful, trusting child's eyes and seeing his innocence drain away as he endures punishment after punishment of the life-giving treatment. And to what end? I know the odds. It is never pretty. It is never a good news story. It is oftentimes not a happy ending.

From today, their family and friends will look on them with sadness, with regret for what might lay ahead. Their calls will be met with tears and disbelief as they let their loved ones into the story of today. First, there will be deafening silence, because there is nothing to say, nothing that will make this chapter of their lives bearable. Then, their well-meaning friends and family will offer platitudes of "It will be okay; everything happens for a reason," or, worse still, "There must be a mistake, the doctors must be wrong, surely this is not truly happening." Finally, they will be called courageous, amazing, resilient, as with every day of their journey, they die a little bit more on the inside, with no choice but to be brave for their precious one. Today their hopes for the future will become single-minded: that their child will survive. There are no more choices; there is only one destination. The dreams of ballet lessons, of perfecting that grand jete; of soccer games and rugby tackles; of being the scientist who makes a world-changing discovery, a world class athlete, or simply the little girl in the blue house – those dreams will evaporate, like their tears, and they will instead begin their nightmare. The kind of nightmare where you can't breathe, no one can hear your scream, and the blessed relief of waking up and discovering it was "just a nightmare" never comes.

I pride myself on being right, I need to be right, I want to be right. But not today. No. I don't want to be right today. I don't want to be the grim reaper that thrusts this little family into dark despair, that pronounces over their lives a journey of heartbreak and pain, with only the smallest glimmer of hope for healing and wholeness. I don't want to be the one who, by uttering those words, dictates a path of pain and suffering for this family. I want to tell them that their little one is fine.

In a few days, their precious son will be back to his usual happy, smiling, and playful self. I want to waltz into their room with my magic wand and bubbles and tell them to go home and enjoy Christmas. Go now, while there is still time for Christmas miracles. Celebrate with your family, none the wiser of what the future might hold. I want to tell them to go home and watch this little one grow. Dream dreams of how their son will change the world.

I don't want to be the one that shatters their dreams, that in a single careful sentence turns their world upside down. Their child has cancer. The computer screen taunts me with the red results, burning into my retina the pathology hidden in the numbers. There is no ignoring this news. I cannot wish it away. I cannot unsee the results. I cannot unhear the pathologist's call and sense of urgency over the phone. My magic wand and bubbles will work no magic today. There will be no giggles or eyes lit with smiles today. Just the descending darkness of grief as the new reality takes hold.

Hope. They need hope. I need hope. Please, God, help me to remain hopeful, always hopeful. To walk alongside strangers and be thrust into knowing them in the most intimate way, in the depths of their despair, as their emotions run raw, and they are forced to face a reality that they didn't choose nor desire to accept – this is my gift. To be allowed into their pain and suffering, their anger and denial, to catch their tears in my hands, even for just a moment, as their story unfolds and a devastating new chapter begins. To share the moment when the walls crash in, the floor falls away, the air becomes too heavy to breathe. I know too well that the words I choose will in some small way change how today unfolds for this family. This is their day one.

I remember my day one. It was different, a different grief, a different journey, but I remember.

I met the man of my dreams at high school. We married and dreamt of a life with a noisy house full of children. Success and joy came in many ways, but our dream of children haunted us. We suffered three early pregnancy losses, our arms and hearts empty and longing for a child. Finally, we were blessed with our precious daughter. How we loved being parents to Stephanie. She was delightful, full of life, and we felt like our world had expanded to absolute joy with her arrival. We were so besotted that we excitedly planned a bigger family.

My husband had coined the term "serial overachiever" for me, many years earlier. It was a term he used with great affection. He was right. I don't like to fail. In fact, I was accustomed to excelling, always excelling. But I had been defeated by my inability to bear children. Our beautiful daughter stole our hearts when she entered our world. But further early pregnancy losses forced us to release our dream of adding to our family. No house filled with noisy children. Time to let that dream go.

Deep down, unattended since leaving high school, was an often stated, always dismissed, burning desire to become a doctor. The disappointment and grief of the loss of our "bigger family dream" kindled the fire for me. In letting go of one dream, another was allowed to surface. No longer a small flicker, the fire in my belly to follow my heart to medicine was fanned into a raging bushfire. I love a challenge!

Medical school it was. I abandoned my life as a Speech Pathologist and headed into the great unknown of medical school. This had become my surrogate second child. My womb might not have been able to carry another child safely into this world, but my sheer determination and grit would mean I could defeat the medical course and, against the odds, become a doctor, even when considered "too old." As vividly as if it were yesterday, I remember my standard reply: "Ah, yes, but I will be old whether or not I study medicine. I will be old whether or not I become a doctor." The running joke was that I needed to live long enough to complete my specialty training. Often, I was forced to resort to the online urban dictionary to be able to participate in the social banter of my young compatriots. My medical school persona was one of mother, confidante, baker, and "crypt keeper." It was not long, in fact, until I resembled the crypt keeper, as the shadows under my eyes deepened and the spring in my step evaporated with the intense, relentless demands of medical school, parenting, and maintaining relationships. Tears of frustration, tiredness, and inadequacy became my familiar companions, but I practiced my mantra: "I am a serial overachiever, and things will be fine."

I settled into a rhythm, formed lifetime friendships, and easily proved to the cynics that I was not "too old" to become a doctor after all. The second year of medical school brought the refreshing change of clinical work, along with the academic load. I loved the opportunity to interact with patients and their families. My practice as a Speech Pathologist had given me excellent skills in communication, and connecting with patients came easily.

Today my day was to begin at Mayne Medical School, a clinical skills tutorial, before we set out to the hospital ward for bedside teaching. Just one more thing before I jumped into the car and headed to my class. I had been fighting a grumbling sense of disquiet over the last week – my period was late. Time to face the music and use that home pregnancy test. It would certainly be negative – too old, too tired for a positive result.

The floor began to fall away as I held myself up on the ice-cold tiles of the bathroom wall. My breathing quickened, and my head started to race. The test seemed to be wilfully provoking me as it became more intense in colour. There was no mistake as I watched the second line appear. My heart leapt into my throat as I fought the rising panic. Gripped with the overwhelming fear of travelling the same road of disappointment, of riding the emotional roller coaster of miscarriage and pregnancy loss, weighed down with the dread of what might come, I didn't tell anyone, not for days, not even my beloved husband.

My mind was crowded with a complex matrix of "what ifs" and "maybes" in the hours that followed. Could I believe things would be different this time? I must believe things would be different. That would be my survival choice. Defying my fears, reframing my thinking, commanding my body to calm, I settled into a routine of acceptance – I was pregnant. I trained myself not to take the darker path, to push away my thoughts of loss, to calm my heart and ignore my disquiet. As time went by, I became quietly optimistic that things would go smoothly this time.

Twenty weeks. I was 20 weeks pregnant, and our baby continued to thrive. I held my breath as I waited for my 20-week morphology scan. I could barely think for the pounding of my heart and the quickening in my breath as we arrived at the sonographer's rooms. The waiting room was crowded, filled with expectant and excited parents. Joyful chatter and laughter drowned out my audibly pounding heart and diverted my attention from my growing fear, convincing me that this time would be different. This time, there would be no disappointment. The ticking clock in the sonographer's room was deafening as we waited for the images to form on the screen. There she was, our precious baby. Kate. Her name would be Kate. My heart leapt with joy in synchrony with her movements as Kate performed somersaults in her private swimming pool. With an unfamiliar bounce to my step and lilt in my voice, I thanked the sonographer for the video evidence of our baby – she was going to have a life beyond my womb.

I was a high-risk pregnancy. I was "elderly" in medical terms, close to my fourth decade, the "crypt keeper," according to my young medical school friends. I sensed my doctor's concern when I had not had any convincing foetal movements as we approached the 24-week mark. Gooseflesh replaced my skin; my stomach dropped to the floor and my body became cold with fear. My legs were like jelly; my eyes burned with tears. I was sure I was going to vomit as I tried to convince myself that there was a foetal heartbeat and movement on the ultrasound screen. Then the darkness closed in. I couldn't breathe, I couldn't make out the words of the sonographer, but her tone – it was the tone of death, disappointment, sadness, as she called for our doctor. The ultrasound screen blurred as my vision narrowed and I clambered into the darkness. No, no, no. Not again. I refused to believe that Kate had died. She was cocooned in the safety of my womb. We had taken home a video of her only four weeks earlier. She had been smiling and waving at us from her secret room. No, no, no. The scan was wrong. My head was spinning, I was going to vomit. What? Go home and wait. Wait. Wait for what? For our baby's birthday to be her death-day? No. I would not accept this. No.

In the days to come, I convinced myself that our doctors were wrong. They didn't have the faith I have; you see, I believe in the God of miracles. Kate was going to change the world. She would survive and her story would be that of a miracle. A wonderful, heart-warming, unbelievable miracle. I worked so hard to unsee her little lifeless body floating in her secret room. I worked so hard to unhear the doctor's words, "I am so sorry. She's dead."

My insides twisted and a thousand knives stabbed my abdomen; my throat was searing in pain, and the heat of tears burned my face. The induction drugs had triggered contractions much sooner than expected. I sat rocking on our hard, icy kitchen floor. I focused on willing Kate to be alive. With every contraction, I was overcome with both physical and emotional pain and anguish. Our baby was coming. This was not how it was meant to be.

"The IUFD[1] is here," the nurse announced. No. No. No. She would not be defined by that label. No! Kate. Her name is Kate. She had been frolicking in her personalised swimming pool, deep in the darkest and safest part of me, just weeks ago. I knew. I had felt the butterfly kisses of her movements, barely detectable but real. From the moment of her conception, Kate's life was precious. Celebrated. From the moment of her conception, we had dreams for her. We knew where she would go to school – she would be there with her sister. Her room was ready. I would not accept this. She would be coming home.

The sterile delivery suite smelled like an operating theatre. There was no mood lighting. No music. Deafening silence, interrupted only by the monitor revealing my racing heart. I couldn't breathe. I couldn't think. The physical pain of Kate's delivery paled as the deep sheering pain of loss swept over me. Without ever taking a breath, without a sound from her tiny body, her tiny perfect body, our baby, Kate, entered the world. Our dreams came crashing down and the darkness descended over us like a thick, dark fog. We held our precious, lifeless Kate and washed her little body with our tears. The nurse came to take her away. "Are you done with her?" My heart exploded with the pain of letting her go. NO! I am not done with her. I am not ready to let her go. I will not send her away. I will not abandon her. I had already failed her once. My body had let her down. I had failed in my primary role as mother to protect her. No. I am not done with her. I will never be done with her.

No amount of determination or grit could change the outcome. We could not unsee or unknow Kate's future. It was time. Time for our precious little one to leave us, before we could even know her. Grief washed over and consumed us as we organised her

---

1 Intrauterine foetal death

funeral – our Kate. It had to be done. There was no choice. There was no easier path. Her birthday was her death-day. We lit a candle to acknowledge her brief little life. There would be no celebration candles. There would be flowers, lots of flowers, but not of celebration.

I could barely lift myself from the bed. My arms and legs were like lead weights. My head, a dark and brooding storm cloud. But there was no time for this. We had a seven year old daughter who deserved better. Stephanie deserved her mumma to be present, to walk alongside her in her grief, to let her in. She couldn't understand the depth of our grief, but she too, had lost a dream. The dream of a baby sister. We needed to grieve together, and life demanded that I find my new normal, that we find our new normal. As if that wasn't enough, medical exams loomed high on the horizon and medical school was demanding a date for my return. My grief continued to paralyse me.

Avoidance of my attendance at medical school was no longer an option, as I was summoned into the Dean's office. There he sat, in his overly large leather office chair, tapping his pen on the polished timber desk. "No." A simple answer. "No. You are a mother. You can do it. You need to do it. I think being a mother should be a prerequisite for medical school. Mothers can do anything they put their minds to." In some backward way, sitting the exams just six weeks after Kate was born was meant to be therapy. I felt the anger rise in me, and I was ready to spew fire in response to these seemingly flippant and unfeeling instructions. Instead, I directed my attention to the narrative running in my head: "Distraction is good, isn't it? Focus. Put your emotions aside. Wear your mask. You are a strong woman. Move on." I pushed my grief down, down, down. My grit and determination again took charge. I wore my mask. I remained silent. Walking out of the Dean's office, I made my decision. I was a serial overachiever, and I would not be defeated.

With the exams behind me, and Kate held closely in my heart, life returned to some semblance of normal, even routine. I excelled at my clinical years and thrived as I approached the finish line. The final months of medical school were clearly on the horizon. I was not too old. I would be a doctor before celebrating my 40th birthday, just. Our family of three were ready for the next chapter. I would soon be heading off to work as a doctor. Then it happened.

A familiar wave of impending doom settled over me as I realised my period was late. Again. Two lines appeared, taunting me like some kind of cruel hoax. Head spinning, fighting for oxygen, the floor beneath me slipping away. This was my eighth pregnancy. I was on the threshold of launching my medical career. Our daughter, Stephanie, was nine years old. Six times we had been dealt the blow of a pregnancy loss. Kate would have been two years old now, if she had survived. Denial was my survival. I would continue on as if this was not happening. I would make no preparations. I would have no expectations. There would be no dreams. I knew the odds. How could I hope for a happy ending?

Alexandra took us by surprise. She entered the world via an emergency caesarean section at 35 weeks. Her cry sounded out through the operating theatre like a jubilant song. I breathed in the perfume of flowers, lots of flowers! My heart was ready to burst with joy at the miracle of our girl's birth. The odds did not determine her future.

***

My bleary eyes open, and my senses are awakened by that delicious smell – nostrils tingling, tummy rumbling, my ears tickled by the sound of sizzling bacon. My beautiful girls, old enough to be just a little independent in the kitchen, have chosen to spoil me this Christmas Eve with an early breakfast, before I head into the Children's Emergency Department. Such a feeling of warmth and fulfillment as they greet me with their exuberant love. Carried away in my moment of mothering bliss, my mouth enjoying the delicacy of crispy bacon and scrambled eggs, prepared in the way only children can, I lose focus of my destination for the day. My enjoyment is cut short as I remember that it is almost time for me to be at work. Handover will begin in a few short moments. I need to be there and engaged, ready to receive the care of those entrusted to me today. My mind wanders as I drive to work, wondering what today will hold.

The tinsel and trees, blinking lights and the smell of freshly baked Christmas shortbread greet my arrival at work. It would be a joyful day. Families would stay home today. The spirit of Christmas has captured the staff as we settle into our morning handover with an unusual sense of joviality. Then, in an instant, the expectation of a joyful day evaporated. I will my eyes to focus on the computer screen. How I wish that the results were wrong.

Not again. I don't want to tell another family that their precious little one has just stepped off a precipice. That their family will soon be plunged into an abyss of agony and pain. That in the minutes to come, they will stand by, watching but unable to control what lies ahead. Not on Christmas Eve, when every family should be filled with the excitement and anticipation that come with Christmas preparations. Not today, when this precious family is about to celebrate their first Christmas with their long-awaited baby.

Please God, let the story be different this time. I want to choose a different outcome for this family. I want the results to be different. I want to be wrong. But no. I am atop the slippery slope, crashing down into the darkness. The floor letting go beneath my feet, my eyes burning, my heart pounding and the air around me like a dark thick cloud, choking me as I try to breathe.

I sit on the bed, and my body sinks into the cool, crisp, sterile sheets with the weight of the conversation to come. I feel like these beautiful young parents look straight into my heart. Every fibre in their beings is willing me to have good news. Patiently they have awaited my return. I have been honest with them at every step. I have shared with them my disquiet. I have been candid with them about the worst-case scenario, wishing with every cell that I would not have to confirm my fears, their fears.

My heart is breaking as I gaze at their little boy. He is perfect. His mop of dark hair tousled out of place. His little fingers grasping his mother's finger. His eyes crystal blue, the eyes of an old soul. Somehow, I sense he knows his future already. I am drawn to his ashen skin, with a smattering of small bruises, the hallmark of his haematological malignancy. The swelling of his leg. There is no denying the truth. My breath catches in my throat. I place my hands on theirs, and as my tears flow, I say, "I am so sorry. The test results confirmed my greatest fear."

With those words, my heart breaks for another family, and I remember. I remember my day one. I remember baby Kate, and I am thankful for my journey. I am thankful that I can know a little of my patients' grief. I am thankful that my heart breaks alongside my patients' family and that I can journey with them, even for a little while.

This is my gift.

CHAPTER 11

Burnt Toast

DR JACINTA PALISE
HOSPITAL STAFF SPECIALIST

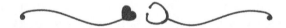

My dearest Jacinta,

Can you even believe that you are finally a doctor?! It has been eight long years of study, copious tears, multiple house moves, and the addition of two adoring dogs and two jerk cats. But you have made it. Firstly, I want to say "congratulations!" because it certainly was an arduous, almost insurmountable journey at times. I mean, certainly, it was rewarding and made you who you are now, but...you were and will continue to be constantly racked by feelings of imposter syndrome, believing that perhaps you aren't smart enough to be a doctor. Deep down, you have that small voice challenging your successes, whispering that you aren't worthy. Looking back now, I have gained some perspective, and I hope to share this with you now, before you enter internship. To prepare you somewhat for the onslaught.

I've had a revelation.

Women are conditioned to think that our self-worth is dependent on our service: what we can do for others. What our bodies look like and can do, as well as our servitude at work and in our homes. This subservience is internalised and so deeply embedded in our sense of self and society that we aren't even consciously aware of it. We are conditioned to believe that we are inferior to our male counterparts in everything we do. And this need to please, this need to serve others, perfectly serves the needs of the men in our lives, our bosses, partners, and colleagues, as we continue to exert ourselves for their satisfaction and pat ourselves on the back for a job well done. For eating our meals over the sink. For serving ourselves the burnt pieces of toast or the steak with all the gristle. For going out of our way to make others comfortable. For putting ourselves last and for perpetuating this internalised, unconscious, misogynistic view that our compliance equals our worth.

Perhaps initially, fueling your own feelings of inadequacy was an event. Years ago, in grade 12, you were involved in a fairly life-altering car accident. I know you will remember this, as it defined your life for a long time; every other occurrence in life could be pinpointed as occurring either "before the accident" or "after the accident". Thankfully no-one died, although, as an overachiever, you did try pretty hard. However, the injuries sustained, including that brain injury, would change your future in other devastating ways.

You died at the scene. You required CPR from a quick-thinking first responder (police-officer Linda, a name forever etched in your soul) who brought you back. You had a bleed on the brain and was flown from your supportive cocoon of a country town to the Big City. On life support, doctors would tell your brother and mum that you will surely die from your injuries, as the swelling in your brain threatened to damage vital, life-sustaining functions. Despite this, however, you would wake, confused and disoriented, and make obnoxious quips to doctors, nurses, and kindly visitors from home. In a regional rehabilitation unit, doctors would give a demoralising prediction: whilst you had lived, the hardest part would be the life-long recovery from the brain injury. A promising career was less likely, with university almost incomprehensible.

Goodness, you were insufferable. You were determined to study science at a university far from home; arguments with your mum would reveal the tension between a headstrong teenager and her protective and – I'll admit it now – **wiser** parent. You compromised and reduced your contact hours, to allow rest and space for healing. An IQ test revealed significantly impaired short-term memory, but you worked hard to pass your exams. It was here that you first experienced biology; you learnt about cells and human anatomy. This first university year, whilst a struggle emotionally, and despite suffering severe, bone-shatteringly profound fatigue, was when you decided to pursue a career in medicine.

A neurologist, reviewing you routinely post-accident, did everything but laugh in your face upon hearing your plan. Sitting there at his expensive, dark timber desk, in his ominous black leather chair, he told you that you wouldn't get into medicine, let alone finish your current degree. But, Jacinta, that stubbornness your family constantly teases you about became the tenacity required to triumph in the face of your critics. It wasn't easy; in fact, college was more like high school than your actual high school experience. You were bullied and humiliated by students, endured at least a few attempted sexual assaults, and were raped once. You woke one night at college, and he was on you. In you. You tried to fight him off, but you were so scared. Paralysed. You dissociated for the rest of it, a protective mechanism to prevent shattering completely. You didn't say anything; who would believe you? Perhaps you hadn't locked your door, or had too much to drink. Maybe you smiled at him once in the mess hall or in a lecture once. Men taking liberties regardless of consent is a theme that will continue in your life, and for women everywhere. You felt ashamed and unsure of who you were and what you were doing; you questioned humanity in the Big City and your aspirations seemed lightyears away at times. But you also met some particularly fabulous humans who will continue as stars in your life, even as I write this. Whilst your path to medicine wasn't easy, it was rich with experience.

Medicine was like nothing you had experienced in undergrad. Still plagued by imposter syndrome, you looked around at those brilliant minds around you and wondered when they would realise that you didn't belong. You cried after almost every exam, sure that this would be the one that unveiled your inadequacies, and cried again when you somehow (miraculously, it seemed) passed. You made some wonderful friends in your small medicine cohort, familiar friendly faces you proudly watched succeed as you moved through your own specialist training. You were consistently supported by your single mum and brother, as well as your boyfriend (newsflash: he proposes!) and his family. You made it through medical school, although still insecure and unsure of who you were, whilst wearing a mask of jaunty exuberance and extroversion. But I promise you, my dear Jacinta, that one day you will no longer feel that you are playing this role; it will feel so natural and real that you know that you belong where you are and who you are with – and you will know who you are. You will finally believe that you are worthy.

In reality, despite graduating from medicine and entering the workforce as an optimistic, wide-eyed intern, I have to tell you that the toughest part is yet to come. That feeling of "worthiness" won't come for some time. To be fair, it isn't your fault. You were born and identify as a woman. However, the world of medicine will make you feel that this one quality is a serious shortcoming.

Proud as punch that you have graduated, you will chat with acquaintances who immediately ask if you are a nurse/ physiotherapist/dietician/naturopath. Now, don't get me wrong, there is certainly nothing wrong with any of those professions but the conversation noticeably stifles when you state that you are a doctor. You have apparently flown in the face of societal convention and made a serious transgression against nature. Whether you notice it or not, men in particular become uncomfortable in conversation, and after a while, you will acquiesce and say that you are indeed a nurse, just to avoid the discomfort and to fulfill this norm. To be fair, you think, the public aren't aware that the vast majority of doctors are female nowadays. and you empathise with the male nurses who must also experience the same. But, my dear Jacinta, have you wondered if this would happen to a man?

Regrettably, it's much the same once you start work and will continue right up to the day I am penning this. You will purposefully introduce yourself as "Doctor Jacinta" in all interactions with patients and their families, often multiple times in opening introductions. Despite this, they will maintain that you are literally any other profession than doctor. You have middle-aged and older male patients refer to you simply using words like "Bub", "Babe", "Baby", "Darling", and "Sweetie", including when they are angry with you. These diminutive terms could be seen as terms of endearment, but really they are a tool utilised to excuse the sexist and inappropriate behaviour which surely follows. You don't ask to be called "Doctor"; hell, you just want to be called "Jacinta" rather than some epithet which permits them to comment on your appearance/youth/womanliness. Once, in the outpatient department, after a 30-minute consultation, a patient will angrily ask when the "real" doctor is coming. In reply, you will emphatically state, attempting to persuade him, that the "real" doctor is, indeed, you; increasingly furious, he will clarify that he means "the real, MALE doctor". Patients and families will constantly and purposefully direct all questions to your less experienced but arguably more "male" colleagues, despite their lack of training and knowledge in your area. You suppose this is to be expected, and it really isn't their fault, as perhaps you are too nice? But, my dear Jacinta, have you wondered if this would happen to a man?

You will start your intern year in a medical specialty you adore, and your consultants will be spectacular! However, sadly, the least assuming and kindest supervisor will ogle you, leaning back to view your silhouette from behind when you greet him one morning. In this moment, you will be frozen and mute, and despite your dimmed smile, you will feel ashamed for wearing that dress. So much so that you won't wear it again. But after all, you wonder, your male colleagues can't be blamed for their innate behaviours, regardless of how it makes you feel. Perhaps the dress was a little too tight, or perhaps you are just being too sensitive. But, my dear Jacinta, have you wondered if this would happen to a man?

You will be the only woman in the surgical team as a junior doctor, and you know that the best offence is a good defence. So, you "play up" the traditional gender role and bake copious cakes and biscuits for the team, whilst ensuring completion of all the paperwork. After all, the other male junior doctor shouldn't really have to do this secretarial job, which is far better suited to a woman. Although this strategy is effective, you do wonder if the team respects you as a clinician. You will quickly dismiss this idea as you remind yourself that the team's male registrar greeted you with a comment that "the way to a surgeon's respect is through his stomach". But, my dear Jacinta, have you wondered if this would happen to a man?

You will have supervisors make sexually explicit comments and jokes, whilst taking your silence as complicity and agreement. Some may mistake this silence as flirtation, despite your discomfort and lack of eye contact. But what can you do? They are your supervisors and you have to pass these rotations. Who would you tell? Who would believe you? It would be your word against theirs, and it would certainly harm your future career; your specialty is very tight-knit, and speaking out would only make life harder. I can tell you now, sweet Jacinta, that throughout your training, you will learn that your experience is not unique; indeed, sexual harassment and discrimination are endemic to our field. The feminisation of medicine over the years has brought this to light, fuelled by sociocultural movements such as #MeToo. Studies will show that the same reasons you don't speak out are the same reasons women in other positions don't. We know that it occurs, but no-one is particularly interested in changing it. You are being an emotional woman and will be blamed for making everything about gender. Perhaps you lead your seniors on by smiling too much or being too personable? But, my darling Jacinta, have you wondered if this would happen to a man?

You will be a junior registrar and be asked to sit with the director of the clinical unit for your mid-semester assessment. This supervisor hadn't spent much time with you, but he will tell you that you needed to be quieter, sit lower than him, and be more passive. This will utterly devastate you. You will hide your tears behind your sunglasses on the train ride home that evening, because the innate personality traits which you believed led to rapport with patients, families, and colleagues had now been described as serious personal and professional failings. Your communication is labelled loud and aggressive, and indeed, if you were a "good" trainee, you would sit quietly and acquiesce to your senior staff, regardless of your opinions or clinical knowledge. These thoughts and comments will fuel your imposter syndrome, and even when you may quietly think you are doing well at a training rotation, you won't be given any such feedback. But, my beloved Jacinta, you will always see comradery between male supervisors and their male registrars, regardless of the latter's clinical competency (or lack thereof).

Things come crashing down when you fall pregnant, rather unexpectedly. But rather than joyously celebrating gestating that precious son of yours, you worry and stew on what this means for your job application the following year. You will cry because you value honesty and need to tell the director at the hospital where you had hoped to work, but doing so will mean that you may not get chosen for a job or burn a bridge for future clinical roles; you will need most of the rotation as maternity leave. You worked with a friend who was constantly bullied whilst pregnant, with both micro and macro aggressions, which wasn't reassuring. Moreover, working on six-month contracts means that the possibility of getting passed over for a job means not receiving paid maternity leave and no income to support your little family. But you realise that you need to make a choice that many women before you have made and many after you will be forced to make; you choose your family over a career and system that does not support women. You start to realise that this certainly isn't a consideration for a man.

It is this experience, my resilient Jacinta, that will be your breaking point. Or perhaps better stated, your rebirth. Oh, don't get me wrong, you will first completely fragment, but will (eventually) put yourself back together until you somewhat resemble the person you were, but different and even perhaps stronger. Like the Japanese art of kintsugi, these cracks are what make you who you are now and potentially more beautiful than you were.

Maternity leave will be a blur. You will hallucinate from sleep deprivation, because your baby won't sleep more than half an hour at a time; this will continue day and night, for weeks and months on end. But as the woman, surely it is your role and your role alone to deal with the night awakenings. After all, you are on holiday.

You don't just magically lose that baby weight, unlike the celebrities who promise that you bounce back within two weeks of birth, and you feel society judging your worth based on that extra 20kg you now carry. You feel that your gender and body fail you; no-one warned that breastfeeding is punishing and not at all a natural behaviour. You and your baby just won't "sync" during this aspect of your relationship that should make you feel like an Earth Mother, nourishing your baby with milk specifically designed for him. No. Instead, your baby will vomit bright red milk, stained with the blood from your bleeding, blistered, and cracked nipples, whilst you are juggling the breast pump and mixing a bottle of formula. Midwives will blame you for starving your baby when he loses 11% of weight when the cut-off for tolerable weight loss in that first week is 10%. How dare your body fail you and

113

your gender seemingly judge you on these failings, whilst they also keep these monumental secrets.

You will wearily return to work when your son is only four months old due to financial constraints. You will cry each time a well-meaning colleague asks who is looking after your baby; it is understood that this is a mother's responsibility, and it appears completely incomprehensible that you would work when there is a more important role to fulfil. Only later will you think of funny quips, like "Oh, I knew I forgot something!" You will express milk at work, three times a day, frantic not to relinquish this one enduring connection with your baby. But you will express in the disability toilet, bone-tired, trying to juggle the bottles so as to not let them touch the floor, and you will cry if and when they do; anyone who says not to cry over spilled milk has obviously not triple-fed due to low supply and dropped that precious breastmilk. You will also weep because it feels that you are simultaneously letting your son down already, as well as your colleagues. You realise, very clearly now, that these occurrences are very specific to the female condition.

Perhaps it is the lack of sleep, or something else intangible that motherhood has awakened, but your tolerance of bullying, discrimination, and sexism will be relegated. Society will allude to the inferiority of womanhood when they say your son screams/ runs/throws like a girl and cannot wear pink. Frustrated, you buy all of the pink clothes from Big W, dressing him exclusively from head-to-toe in unicorns and love hearts and rainbows and flowers. In doing so, however, you notice that the "girl" toddler shorts are several inches shorter than those in the "boy" section; society sexualises women from such a young age. All of the frills and dresses we buy our little girls must surely hold them back in playing and inform them that, as women, we should be passive and clean and feminine. That society values women who look and dress a certain way. Shouldn't little kids run, jump, and fall, without showing off their underwear? Shouldn't we tell little girls that their worth is more than what they wear and what they look like? You can start to see how your beliefs about your self-worth, your body, and your appearance will begin to change.

You will see your life, your career, and your teaching in a new light. You will no longer apologise for being a woman and know absolutely that your strength comes from this exact characteristic.

Your kindness will not be mistaken as weakness. You will no longer stand by when patients or family members call you or your staff those names, or comment on your clothes/body/weight/face/make-up/lack of make-up/smile. You will remind them, politely but assertively, that you and your staff deserve to feel comfortable at work and that sexually suggestive comments will not be tolerated. You will do this pointedly in front of your female juniors to set a standard, whilst emphatically educating the males so that they will (hopefully) not be ignorantly complicit to such behaviours.

Teaching will bring vigour to your day, but you will be saddened by a story recounted by a female medical student. She narrates a conversation with a male surgeon who once told her that she could not simultaneously have a successful career, a happy marriage, and well-adjusted children; she would have to choose only two. As a result, she gave up on the notion of a neurosurgical career, dissuaded intentionally or not by this male supervisor in an unspoken power differential. Just imagine, the entire life of a person changes with just one statement made, perhaps offhandedly. Perhaps it speaks to a sad truth that women aren't supported enough in their training. This medical student was knowledgeable, compassionate, and driven; she could have pioneered a new surgical technique, struck fame and fortune, or perhaps even more importantly changed the lives of her patients and their families. But in one conversation, she was told that she was never going to be "enough". Interestingly, that surgeon was a father and a husband and had a career; perhaps the rules are different for men.

Another medical student would comment with such resignation at the end of her rotation with you that she knows she shouldn't be "too" confident. She elaborates that confident women are seen as "bitchy", whilst confident men are revered. You would spend some time with this student so that she knows that she can be confident and kind, and that the traits exhibited by men can be matched by women, but that we need to change the conversation. Supervisors often speak about the emotional traits of female trainees in their end-of-term reports; women are often compassionate and good communicators, which does not necessarily speak to confidence, competence, and knowledge. You will feel disheartened, as you know certainly that these conversations do not occur between male doctors.

At a teaching course, you will sit and reflect on the imposter syndrome that has followed you for years, like debt or herpes. Women around you, brilliant minds in allied health, medicine, and nursing, will nod all-knowingly along with your stories and experience, as if this was a secret that all women must carry, a feeling of inadequacy in your role despite performing it with compassion, wisdom, and vigour. Further proving your unspoken belief, the male course convenor, a prominent lecturer and clinician at this prestigious university, will state that surely this feeling, this feeling of being an imposter in your own life and role, demonstrates a struggling, even underperforming clinician; he could not begin to comprehend this feeling because it appears his innate maleness prevented it. You will look around and see similar questions and incomprehension in many other men's eyes, whilst simultaneously noting the sadness and awareness in your female colleagues. Whilst I want you to appreciate that this is not uniquely a female experience, as you have come to recognise it in some of your male trainees who are high performing with significant emotional intelligence, it is far more ubiquitous in female professionals.

You will continue to see inequality in everything: at work, at home, and in society. Over the years, you will hear what seems like the same story from all your female friends: the significant mental and physical load of being married, of having a family, of endless housework and cooking after finishing work. You will feel both helpless and inexhaustibly fuelled by the desire to raise your son and your junior staff into a different world. One where #MeToo is a distant memory, and the gender pay gap no longer exists. One where women are not victim-blamed for wearing a skirt, drinking alcohol, or being out after dark, but where instead men are held accountable for their actions. A world where the mental load is shared amongst partners, and women are supported in their training, pregnancy, and breastfeeding, and wholeheartedly supported in reintegration into the workforce. You will also, perhaps most importantly, recognise your own privilege as a white, cis-gendered, heterosexual woman, and that many others who do not fit these "norms" are continually in receipt of worse attacks; you will make it your daily goal to stand up for yourself and others.

You will reflect on your experiences, as a victim of sexual assault, and your interactions with males in a position of power, who will be sexually suggestive whilst you feel powerless. You will reflect on your cognitions about walking in the dark at night if you finish work late, watching for movement which might represent an impending attack. You have been told that you are "too loud", "too nice", "too trusting", "too tall", "too smart", "too mature" and "too much" at various points in your life, but you will (eventually) come to realise that you are enough. You will realise that when complaints are made by your male colleagues, this is because you did not passively bend to their will and instead respectfully shared an opinion that differed from their own; how dare you! You will be asked to smile more (which is your innate default), and if you aren't smiling due to stress or an overly active mind filled with the mental load, you will be asked if you are angry or have insinuated that you are overwhelmed and underperforming. It appears that society views a woman's worth and role as constantly being busy: to work as if she doesn't have a family, and to provide for her family as if she doesn't work. But, my impassioned Jacinta, you will just. Not. Care. You will focus on your patients and their families, advocating for them, your colleagues, and your unit. You will be professional and respectful and care for your trainees and students. You will do what you can for your gender, whilst walking the political tightrope to not piss off too many bosses. You will know that you are worth the air that you breathe and life that you possess. You will know that your femininity and "womanliness" are essential to your strength, including your high heels, which have purportedly scared some men.

You don't hate men, but you will learn to approach interactions and relationships with them with weariness, for too often they have taken liberties with your body and ideas. No, you don't hate men; you love your husband and adore your son, and have many positive relationships with men in your life. But you will also come to realise, my resilient Jacinta, that out of all your relationships, your relationship with yourself deserves the most profound love and respect. Only then can and will you work to rid yourself of society's conditioning. It won't be easy, but it will be worth it. Because you are worth it.

WE are worthy.

Anyway, I better be off to fight the good fight. I might burn a bra later, or perhaps bake a cake. And I'll definitely do it wearing glittery heels and reclaiming my title of "feminist". Whatever I do, I know that the choice is entirely mine. Life is crazy and bright and beautiful. You are lucky to be alive. So go on, make it worth it. Wreak havoc.

Warmest regards in feminism and passion,

Dr. Jacinta

Feminist, doctor, wife, teacher, mother, daughter, sister, friend, boss.

P.S. Your son still doesn't sleep. You sort of get used to it. Kinda.

CHAPTER 12

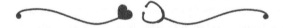

DR MOKGOHLOE TSHABALALA
OBSTETRICIAN & GYNAECOLOGIST

"In resuscitating a pregnant woman in a quest to save mom and perhaps baby too, what item do you need to perform a perimortem caesarean section?"

The sea of blank faces in the lecture theatre was a clear indication that the group of junior registrars had no idea of the response the lecturer was looking for. We all failed to come up with one correct answer. Several of us mentioned various operating tools and drugs. To narrow the list to one thing seemed impossible.

"A sterile blade is all you need," said the consultant, pleased with himself.

It is an introductory question he asks each time he gives this lecture. One hundred percent of the time, students get the answer incorrect, year in and year out. Each time, when he finally gives away the answer, almost all students are dissatisfied with the answer. Almost always, the zealous and confident students raise their hands with questions that attempt to challenge this. He answers all questions, dismissing the importance of all other tools. "A sterile blade", he repeats, in the manner a father speaks to a child, to put a matter to bed.

Year in and year out, students leave that lecture dissatisfied, me included. My dissatisfaction was that, if you have a blade, with a single stroke, one cuts all the layers of the abdominal wall until one reaches the target organ, the womb. Another stroke to the womb, a baby is born, but then what? What do you use to repair that very womb and the abdominal wall that now has severed vessels bleeding the very life out of the patient? Surely one cannot suture with a blade. One needs suture material. Suture material would be crucial.

I had courageously put my hand up, to challenge the lecturer. This was not easy for me, considering how incredibly shy I was as a student. Perhaps shy is a lazy description of how I was, and one that is well accepted in society. I was not shy; I was engulfed by imposter syndrome, and it had not lifted throughout my undergraduate degree. Failing anatomy class and having to repeat it for a whole year did very little to uplift this syndrome. As a matter of fact, it may have worsened it. University swallows one whole, preying on the ones with poor self-esteem the most.

A large crowd of students in an auditorium compared to a mere twenty pupils in a class in high school often left me paralysed with anxiety and my voice often squeaked each time I spoke, so I avoided it as much as I could. I spoke only when spoken to – but not on that day. That day I was confident that my question would settle this matter once and for all.

The confidence must have been evident even in the manner I shot my hand up from beneath the table. I even clicked my fingers to get his attention. His eyes met mine and he acknowledged me. I stood, which was not at all necessary; we could speak seated, but I wanted to be audible and clear.

Professor Hoosein asked, "What is your name, young lady?"

"Refilwe Monaheng, sir," I replied. My voice did not squeak. It was clear and powerful.

"Aaah, Dr Monaheng, you have a question?" Prof asked.

My confidence was now bordering on arrogance I did not know I had. I stood chest out and chin up. "Prof, surely one cannot repair a wound with a blade. One needs a suture material." Professor Hoosein was not at all moved by my challenge. It seemed that over the years, others must have suggested the same. He used his masculine stature – height, broader shoulders, and a deep voice – to overpower me. He stood near and above me like a tower; I could even smell his aftershave. He answered, "The definition of a caesarean section is delivery of a foetus through the incision of the abdominal wall and the uterus. Repairing the uterus after a caesarean section is exactly that – repairing the uterus. And for that, yes –," he held out his index finger to reinforce his point, "– one does need a suture material."

My confidence and arrogance shrank from a pine tree in the forest to a shrub in the desert. I quickly assumed my "speak when spoken to" persona.

As dissatisfied as I was, and as were all my classmates, throughout our training we all learnt to answer that question in that manner each time a lecturer asked – a sterile blade. And so, it went on; every now and then a new lecturer would ask, whether in a tutorial, oral exam, or written exam. We gave that ideal answer, bit our tongues to what each one of us in their heart of hearts believed was the necessary tool, and moved swiftly along. The answer rolled out easily on our tongues, though a silent protest for me was suture material, others, alcohol to disinfect the skin before incision, others an assistant surgeon, and so on.

One time I had to answer that question, which somehow popped up every so often in my training, was when it mattered the most – on a Thursday morning a day before Good Friday.

As doctors, we are always wary of an empty high-care at handover, especially if you are the doctor taking over. It is almost always too good to be true. It's nature's way of preparing for the storm ahead. On that fateful Thursday, I arrived to start my shift to an empty high-care. The high-care ward was an eight-bed unit, designed and equipped for high-risk maternity cases. At any given time, it was fully occupied by sick pregnant or postpartum women, separated from their new-borns to allow their bodies to recover from the trauma of labour or c-section complications. This time around, the unit was quiet, no machines beeping to alert the health care worker to something or another going wrong. The beds were neatly made with crisp white hospital linen, waiting for their next occupant. There was one patient in the active phase of labour, progressing well on the partogram in the labour ward. The foetal monitor attached to her gravid abdomen and the screen by her side recorded a healthy foetal heart rate pattern.

She lay on the hospital bed going in and out of sleep, woken by each contraction. Although this was an ideal handover round, experience had taught me better; I knew this was the calm before the storm, which left me rather unsettled.

I released my colleague once the ward round was done and settled down in the doctors' rest room. This was a little room in a building opposite the labour ward. It was fitted with a single bed, a desk with a lamp, and a shower on its right. All these facilities we seldom utilized, as there was never time to nap or study, let alone shower, on a 24-hour shift. I checked my phone to ascertain that, one, it was not on silent, and two, that I had not missed a call from the midwife in the labour ward.

Exactly forty-five minutes into the calm, the storm hit.

"Dr Monaheng, we have a 17-year-old Palesa Mkhwanazi. She is a primigravida at term in the latent phase of labour, presenting with mild hypertension, escorted by the paramedics and family. Doc, she seems out of breath."

That was the nurse in admissions calling me through the switch board. The general rules you learn when a nurse calls you: one, not to panic, because most nurses exaggerate symptoms; two, not to ignore a nurse when she calls you. They also often underestimate the presentation of the patient. In less than five minutes, I was in admissions. The three-minute walk from the restroom managed to increase my heart rate at least twofold. I needed to calm myself down, but there was just no time.

I had been summoned to an emergency countless time before. As a doctor, you march right into one, assess the severity of the situation in seconds, and begin to reverse the ailing body from a pathological state to a physiological state. We are trained to work and think on the spot and to be systematic so that we don't miss a thing. This time was different. I felt my face heating up beneath my skin, my palms clammy with sweat. I was terrified to walk into that resuscitation bay. Given a choice of fight or flight, I would have fled, but I marched right in. On arrival, Palesas' condition was nothing like what the nurse described; she looked much worse. Either she had deteriorated dramatically in the five minutes it took me to get to her, or the nurse had underestimated her clinical condition. A woman stood by her side, who I assumed was her mother. She wore a black beret, a red jersey, and a black pleated skirt that went down to her ankles. With one hand, she stroked Palesa's forehead, whispering inaudible words; her facial expression urged her to respond, but she did not. She had rolled up the sleeves of her jersey, exposing bracelets made of animal hide on her wrists. I made a mental note that the family may have sought alternate medicine before coming to us. In her other hand, Palesa's mom held a carton of banana flavoured Mageu. Mageu, a carbohydrate-loaded viscous drink made of maize meal, is often used as a home remedy for an unwell and weak person. She had been trying to make Palesa drink it prior to the ambulance arriving at their home. Yet another thing to make a note of, she is pregnant, and with a potentially full stomach. The odds will be against me should I need to intubate her.

By now Palesa was air hungry, breathing twice as much as an ordinary pregnant woman would. Her air hunger state was making her uncooperative; she pulled the oxygen mask off her face and pulled out the intravenous line that the nurses had put up on arrival.

"Call the intern, call the medical officer, and get the resuscitation trolley now!" These were my orders to the nurse. "Get the family out of here!" It will later haunt me, how I screamed for them to leave the room. That was the first impression I made on them, at their most vulnerable moment. I must have made them feel that they were in the way.

With the poly-mask tight against her face, oxygen was at 10L per minute. "Palesa, breathe in and out," I said. She was now kicking violently; her chest sounded like someone rubbing two raw edges of styrofoam against each other. She had pulmonary oedema, a deadly complication of hypertension in pregnancy, where one's lungs are drowning in fluid.

"Eighty milligrams of furosemide!" I yelled.

"In, Doc," the nurse said, to indicate the orders were heard and the medicine administered.

The patient wasn't responding. "Palesa. Palesa! Damn it! Still no response. The monitors attached to her recorded a slow heart rate, no blood pressure, and her skin was turning a dusky blue colour.

"She is going to arre..."

I did not complete the sentence, because her heart stopped. "Hard board behind her back, start CPR," I said to the team. The medical officer jumped on to her chest and thrust on her precordium to restart her heart. With the endotracheal tube ready, just as I was about to intubate her, copious Mageu secretions in her airway occluded my view. The thrusting of her chest to bring the heart back unfortunately presses with the same vigour on her stomach, bringing the stomach contents up to the airway.

"I can't see the cords; I can't see the vocal cords! Suction!" I yelled to the sister.

I suctioned the airway and got a partial view of the vocal cords, which was enough for me to intubate her, but between the unsteadiness of my then-shaking hands from the adrenalin in my bloodstream and the constant up and down movement of her chest from the chest compressions, conditions to intubate were suboptimal. I managed to discipline my right hand, which was holding on to the laryngo-scope, and got into the rhythm of the movement of her moving chest. An opportunity presented itself, so I intubated her successfully and secured the ET-tube with a tape prepared by the student nurse. Mechanical ventilation, chest compression, repeated boluses of adrenalin ensued. But we couldn't seem to get Palesa back. Not even the defibrillator managed to give us a workable rhythm for her heart again.

"A sterile blade," I thought out loud. Within seconds, my mind left the room. In my mind, I was back in Professor Hoosein's lecture hall many years ago. Time froze, albeit for a moment.

"Get me a sterile blade," I repeated, back in the resuscitation bay.

With the intern at her airway and the medical officer and the senior-most sister taking turns on chest compressions, I moved over to Palesa's abdomen. With the sterile blade in my left hand, I answered the question, only that time I was convinced that this was all I needed to perform a perimortem caesarean section. Two strokes, one on the abdominal wall, a second on the womb, and then I handed the blade safely over to the sister. I asked for fundal pressure; an alive, 3.4 kg male baby was born, barely breathing, with a weak pulse and a dusky blue colour all around – but alive. The baby was handed over to the nursery staff and the paediatrician to commence resuscitation of the new-born. All this time, resuscitation was ongoing for mom as well, but Palesa was not coming back. I was given suture material that the sisters kept in the labour ward to repair episiotomies after a normal vaginal delivery. I repaired the uterus. Twenty-five minutes later, we "called it" – medical language, meaning to stop resuscitation and certify the patient dead. I finished off closing the skin, removed gloves, washed my hands, and meticulously recorded all events in the patient's bed letter. A very important step, because it is not ordinary that a 17-year-old dies so suddenly. When they do, in desperation fingers are pointed and should have, could haves are said. Everyone involved must give a detailed account, and rightly so. I ended the notes in the bed letter with time of death, 17:45, stating the cause thereof, and time of delivery, 17:35, and circumstances thereof. I walked out of admissions to go face the family and break the sad and good news. But first, I made a pass to the nursery, to see and explain to the one that deserved an explanation the most, baby to Palesa Mkhwanazi, born: 2nd April 17:35. That was how his name tags read on his ankles. I found him sucking on his bottom lip, pink, full of life and oblivious to what had just taken place. Tears in my eyes, I communicated with him silently. *We tried so hard to save you both, but we couldn't. I'm sorry, baby, Mom didn't make it.*

Perhaps it would have been better to leave you in your mom's belly, never to be separated but to die with her, instead of a life that you are now going to face without a mother. All this time, I had my left pinkie wrapped in his right hand. Just as I let his hand go, I thought I felt a squeeze, or did I imagine it? Our eyes locked on to each other in a long gaze. Did I imagine that, too? The moment was interrupted by a nurse coming towards us, saying he was due for a feed. I left the nursery with a heaviness in my heart, to face the family that was now in the counselling room. Although there were chairs provided for in the room, nobody was seated. I offered them a seat; they declined.

"Re tla ema Mme -ngaka," her mother said, which directly translated means "We prefer to stand, mother-doctor." Mme -ngaka is a respectable way that female doctors are addressed in Sesotho. After ordering them out of the resuscitation bay the way I did, I felt unworthy of the title Mme-ngaka.

With all the commotion, they must have known that something was not right. I broke the news as trained, with all of us on our feet as per their request. Palesa's mom took off the beret on her head and covered her face with it; she turned her back to all of us and let out a wailing cry that came out straight from her core, resulting in what felt like a fine tremor in the room.

I went on to say: "We did everything we could to save mom and baby." I gave them space to grieve as a family and went to the doctors' room. Once the door was locked behind me, I grabbed the pillow, hugged it tight to my chest. I let go and sank to the floor, my back against the door. With my face buried in the pillow, I too let a wailing cry of despair and agony escape my core. I let it out and hoped and prayed that the pillow would catch it all, muffle the sound and make it inaudible to a passer-by.

Two days later, the family came back. This time, Palesa's mom wore a black head scarf and a black jersey with the same black pleated skirt, exposing her ankles, which appeared thinner than the first time I'd seen her. She wore a blanket over her shoulders secured by a large safety pin over her chest, clothes of mourning. She was surrounded by an entourage of women in similar apparel and men in tartan winter blazers despite the warm weather, hats, and wooden sticks. They requested to be given a private moment in the room, by the bed that Palesa died in. We allowed them. We drew the curtains behind them, to give them privacy but still allow clinical activities to continue in the ward for other patients. This is a ritual practiced by many African cultures, to fetch the spirit of the deceased, to take it home.

They came with an undertaker to collect the body and spirit of their child, and a baby car seat to collect their new addition to the family from the paediatric ward.

It has been seven Good Fridays since that fateful one, and many other devastating outcomes, too many to journal about, too many to keep track of their anniversaries, but I often wonder how life panned out for baby Palesa Mkhwanazi, born motherless. I wonder, did their spirits connect as one crossed over to life and another to death? Were they at least afforded a mother and son moment just before she departed? In that spiritual moment, did Palesa pass to her son all that he would need to navigate a world without a mother?

CHAPTER 13

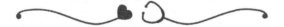

HELEN ZAHOS
EMERGENCY NURSE AND PARAMEDIC

Watarru Clinic, Remote South Australia

Oh fuck, I'm dead. The axe came flying past my face and embedded in the chocked-open door.

It all happened in slow motion.

I stared at the axe in the door with disbelief. I turned to where it had come from and saw a large, dark figure standing in the doorway of the health clinic – it was an Indigenous man. My eyes were wide open, taking in everything that was happening, and I tried to focus on the figure standing there. The bright sunlight behind him made it difficult for me to see, but I soon made out his facial features and his thin, patchy, unkept beard. It was Billy. He was so tall and muscular that he looked like a rugby player, heavyset and stocky. His body filled the frame of the doorway to the cage that enclosed the front area of the clinic and served as an additional barrier to protect the clinic's staff.

His chest was puffed out and he held a spear in his hand. From somewhere deep inside him, he gave out a deafening roar and then started yelling in the Pitjantjatjara language. I had heard this sound before, when there was a dispute between rival clan members. Witnessing it, the sound alone made your heart stop. It was tribal and it meant war. His piercing eyes produced such anger; he took a deep breath, and then yelled even louder, with absolute rage. He raised his arm up and made a fist with his free hand – the one he had just used to throw the axe with – and then punched the cage. The cage shook and vibrated as he hit it again. With his other hand, he raised the spear and pointed it towards me, continuing to yell.

This is it, I'm dead. I've got no fucking way out.

I was frantic. I looked past him at my car, parked outside. He was blocking my only exit.

I didn't even make a noise. You would think I'd scream or yell out for help, but nothing came out of my mouth. I wanted to scream, but I felt winded, like I'd been hit in the stomach.

The Watarru Store

Earlier that morning, I had gone across to the store to get something to eat.

Behind the counter at the store, there was a middle-aged man with red hair that I had never seen before.

'You must be new?' I said. He looked a little anxious or unsure of himself.

'I'm Kevin, yeah, just filling in for the store manager after what happened last week,' he said to me, almost whispering in case someone else in the store heard him.

'Ah,' I said. 'Kevin, he is just outside.' I acknowledged what he was saying with a nod and pointed towards the front door. 'Yes, I heard that he terrorised some people with a star picket and they fled in a hurry. Don't worry, he seems okay. He's sitting outside with his grandmother.'

He smiled at me and pointed to my arm. 'What happened to your arm? Looks nasty.'

I looked down at my bandaged right forearm.

'Oh!' I said. 'You wouldn't believe it; I got bitten by a dingo on Friday. It's a long story, but the vet asked me to help put down "Lucky," the dingo that lives near Pipalyatjara. He'd been sick for some time and was suffering, but as I finished injecting him he jumped up so suddenly and knocked me over and came for my face, so I put my arm up to protect myself and he bit me. I don't blame him, poor thing. The bandage is a bit much but I wanted to keep it covered out here while I was working in the clinic.' I casually took a sip of Diet Coke from the can.

'That is unreal,' Kevin said. 'I can't believe what you nurses have to do out here, hey.'

'Yeah, I even had to sedate a horse once, but that is a story for another day!' I winked at him as I walked out of the store and headed towards the clinic.

I saw Billy was still sitting with his grandmother. There were two women sitting on the ground around a fire outside the front of their house, making wood carvings and burning patterns into them with a wire they were heating up in the fire. The women wore brightly coloured dresses that really stood out beautifully against their skin. I nodded my head to say hello. They both nodded back and one yelled out, 'Nyuntu Palya Kunga?' I smiled and waved and said, 'Palya.' I had developed a fondness for this community.

I approached Billy and his grandmother Gloria, wary of the reports of the previous week. I said hello to both of them, but only Gloria nodded and said hello back to me. She had tired and resigned eyes. Billy stared straight ahead; he was stoney-faced and did not acknowledge me. He sat cross-legged in the red dirt and continued to stare straight ahead. I was not going to try too hard to interact with him on the off chance he reacted badly. I spoke to Gloria and politely said that I had a message from the doctor that Billy was due to have his monthly injection.

'Owa palya', said Gloria in a soft voice. 'He will come to the clinic after lunch, palya?'

'Palya,' I replied, smiling. 'I will see you later, Billy, when you are ready.' I walked away, feeling like half of a difficult job was done. I took in the last little bit of sun on my face and smelt the smoke in the air, blowing across from the nearby campfire, and stepped back into the clinic.

Child's Play

I had to finish cleaning the clinic, wiping down surfaces and putting sheets in to wash, and then prepare my things to pack up and go. I continued mopping the floors and spinning the blood samples. The pathology for the laboratory would be collected on the Friday plane that came out to Pipalyatjara once a week to drop off the mail. While I was finishing up the mopping, I heard a clunk on the cage of the clinic. I didn't take too much notice. Sometimes it was the children playing outside, throwing things, that would hit the cage.

Clunk.

There it was again. Definitely someone out there. *Those little shits!* I thought to myself. *Why are they not in school?* As I looked at my watch, I remembered it was school holidays. *Of course the children will be bored, and I bet it's the kids throwing rocks at the clinic.* Watarru was one of my favourite communities in the APY lands that I had been sent to work in as a remote area nurse.

Clunk.

There it was again. I started to walk towards the door, already giggling on the inside that I was sneaking up on the kids, to playfully yell at them as if I were telling them off. They never took me seriously, anyway. It didn't help that I would be laughing as I did it. They often ran up to me so I could pick them up and lift them into the air, or high fived me as they walked into the clinic, skipping along, smiling and showing me white teeth that looked even whiter against their brown skin.

Clunk.

I crouched low, so as not to be seen through the window. My usual trick was to stick my head out the door and playfully yell, 'Right! What is going on here?' The children would giggle and wave or pretend to run away, and then return, laughing in anticipation of what I would do next. As I approached the door, I was ready to call out with a smile on my face, but I couldn't see any children outside. Oh, I thought. *They must have moved down towards the store, the cheeky rascals.* I stood up straight and stepped out into the cage to see if I could see them. It was at that moment the axe came flying past my face.

***

I stood there, paralysed, staring at the spear raised at my head. Finally, I managed to muster up a move and stepped backwards into the clinic. I had both my hands raised up, palms open in a surrender pose. I looked at the bandage on my right wrist. It began to throb, and I began to feel even more vulnerable. Suddenly, I hoped that the bandage would buy me some time, that Billy would take pity on me and not harm me. I glanced at the axe in the door with a helpless feeling and started to go into survival mode. I kept moving back slowly, looking left and right for ways out, planning for what I could use to defend myself. His yelling continued. As he made his way to the doorway, he grabbed the axe with his free hand and pulled it out of the door. With a threatening gesture, he raised the axe above his head, ready to throw again.

I moved backwards slowly, down to the back of the clinic and towards the pharmacy door. I reached for the handle behind me and pushed down on it. It wouldn't move. The door was locked. I raised my hands in front of me again, palms open, and showed him my already wounded arm. Was he really going to hurt me? Or was he just threatening me?

As I thought it, he swung his right arm back with the axe and catapulted it in my direction. I didn't need to move, as the axe fell short of hitting its target, landing on the ground at my feet. I stared at the axe, but before I could even comprehend what had happened, Billy stormed forward and picked it up off the ground. Now he towered above me. I could smell his pungent underarm odour. He was unkept and didn't bathe frequently. I was backed up against the wall, with no way out. I stood there, watching his body; I was not going to go down without a fight. With an inner strength I never knew I had, I calmly spoke, without a hint of the fear I was feeling.

'Billy, it's okay. I'm not going to hurt you. Let's talk about what is going on.' I couldn't read him. He didn't seem to hear what I said. His dark brown eyes seemed even darker with his dilated pupils. *I don't think I can reason with him.* Billy continued glaring at me with those scary eyes. He raised the spear even higher, ready to throw it. He aimed it at my throat and yelled at me again in the Pitjantjatjara language with a menacing look on his face.

The words were ones I didn't recognise. *What was he saying?*

'Billy, I can't understand what you are saying.'

Again my voice was calm and unwavering, even though on the inside I was trembling. 'Please, let's just talk and you can tell me what the problem is and why you are upset.'

Billy started taking in deep breaths and puffing his chest out again, and with each exhalation I waited to see if he would say anything.

And then it happened. He yelled out in English.

'I don't want that fucking needle!' he bellowed in a heavy Aboriginal English accent.

A high-pitched scream followed his statement.

Was that it? Was he serious? All of this so he wouldn't have to have his antipsychotic injection? I was almost relieved, because at least now I could somehow reason with him.

'Billy, you don't have to have the injection if you don't want to. Just go,' I said, exasperated. I waited, still watching his body. *One step forward and I'm going in. I'm not going down without a fight.* I reminded myself of the plan because I wasn't out of danger yet.

Suddenly, he moved. I was ready to pick up a nearby chair and step forward, but then, instead of taking a step towards me, he took a step back. I hadn't thought of that scenario. He lowered the axe and the spear, turned around, and started to walk towards the front of the clinic.

Clunk.

He tapped the blunt part of the axe against the cage as he walked through.

Clunk.

He tapped the axe on the cage again, toying with me. He had a child-like grin on his face, as though he had gotten his way, and casually stepped out of the cage and walked away. I waited a minute, until he was out of sight, and then ran out and closed and locked the cage door.

'P' for Police

I looked at the telephone, on the wall next to the workbench. A list of phone numbers was taped on the wall. I had to call the police and needed their satellite telephone number. My hands were trembling as I traced down the list of numbers with my finger. The week earlier I had asked one of the Aboriginal health workers, Mary, to rewrite and update the phone list.

I had a soft spot for Mary. She was my friend. We often went for walks around Watarru rock, which was also called Mt. Lindsay. Mary had shown me old Indigenous paintings on the side of the rock that were made long before her grandmother's time. This place was sacred.

I stared at the phone list, at Mary's handwriting, and found the word 'police.' I dialled the number on the satellite phone. I felt flustered and in shock; it was as if the adrenaline had gone and my legs were giving out under me. I had never experienced this before. I was normally so strong, but my heart was now racing. I suddenly felt nervous and didn't know how to start explaining the story to the police.

'Hello?' A male voice answered the phone on the other end.

I could hear my voice wavering and I started to cry. 'Hi, it's Helen. I'm a nurse calling from Watarru clinic.' I took a shaky breath and waited.

The voice on the other end unexpectedly sounded jovial. 'G'day, Helen, how's it going?' he said in an overly familiar way. I was surprised and relieved. He sounded like he knew me, so I started rambling. There was no beginning, no middle, and no end; the message was garbled.

'Billy came into the clinic and threw an axe at me and I was bailed up and he trashed the place and now he is outside but I don't know where he is and I'm locked up in the clinic and what if he decides to burn the clinic down with me in it?' My legs finally gave way and I sank to the ground, aware of the freshly mopped floor. A clinic had been burnt down in Ernabella two years earlier, so that was playing in the back of my mind. I sat on the floor and kept filling in the details, as if any minute I was going to die and this was my only chance to speak. Then, just as I thought I had painted a good picture and was relieved because I'd been able to hold it together enough to tell the story, there was a pause at the other end of the line. It was as if the policeman was trying to process the story.

'Alright, Helen,' he said finally. 'Listen to me, you just hang on tight. Stay inside the clinic. I'll close up the pool, round up some of the fellas, and we are on our way!'

Right then, my heart sank. The pool? Close the swimming pool? Oh, no, it was Jason, the pool man, who had taken a liking to me and hinted he wanted to go out sometime.

I quickly looked at the numbers on the wall and saw that Mary had written down the numbers incorrectly on the phone list. I hadn't rung the police; I had rung the swimming pool.

'Oh, no, Jason, it's okay. Don't worry, I'm trying to call the police.' I couldn't hide my disappointment.

'Oh, that's okay,' he said. 'I can see them across the road at the store. Do you want me to go flag them down? You might not be able to get through to their satellite phone? I'll race over quickly! Okay?' He sounded eager to assist and come to my rescue.

'Please, Jason, can you tell them to come quick?' I asked, knowing I could trust him to do this one task and pass on the message. I reached out and put a shaky line through the word 'police' with a black pen and changed it to 'pool.'

A Grandmother's Love

While I waited for the police to arrive, I finished packing my overnight bag in the clinic's back room where I slept when I was on the clinic circuit. I heard a gentle tap on the cage. I yelled, 'The clinic is closed!' Frustrated, because I knew I couldn't ignore whoever it was, I walked towards the front door and peered through the window. It was Billy's grandmother, Gloria. She had such a gentle nature; I knew that I was safe and she was not here to cause problems.

'Sorry, Pampa, I didn't realise it was you!' I exclaimed, smiling at Gloria. I wanted to show her that I was okay with her and that her grandson's actions hadn't changed anything between us.

'Kunga, I found this.' She pulled the axe from under her long skirt; the spear she held like a walking stick. Billy must have left them at the house. I unlocked the cage door, opening it slightly; I was suddenly scared to chock it open like usual. Gloria passed the axe and spear through the gap in the door, and then reached her arm through and gently pressed her palm on my forehead, as if I were sick and she was checking for a fever. She looked down at the ground in shame, unable to look at me. 'Munta.' It was such a small word, but it was so powerful. Right then I wanted to embrace her.

'You don't have to say sorry!' I exclaimed. 'This is not your fault, Gloria! Palya?' She was the sweetest grandmother.

'Do you know where he is? Are you safe? Do you want to come inside the cage and hide?' I was worried for her safety.

'Wiya,' she said 'Palya, Billy is over there, near the big tree. He has his belt and is saying bad things.' She gestured to the other side of the community, with a worried look on her face, like only a grandmother would that loved her grandchild despite his actions.

'What kind of bad things is he saying?' I asked.

She whispered it, as if saying it out loud would make it come true. 'He says he is going to hang himself.' With that, she turned and started to walk away, her shoulders hunched and her head bowed. I watched Gloria disappear behind some houses. I could sense how sad and troubled she was by her grandson's behaviour and the shame she would have felt in the community.

If You Can't Hack It

I heard a troopy pull up. The diesel engine made a distinct noise. It was the police. After four hours, they had arrived. I didn't quite know what to do. Should I go outside and meet them? I felt like I was no longer in danger and I felt like a fool now for having called them. I was embarrassed, as I didn't know where Billy was, and I was still in disbelief and shock. I didn't want to waste their time, but if they arrested Billy now, they would have to drive 16 hours to get him to Alice Springs.

I unlocked the cage door so they could come in. I didn't wait for them and went back inside. Help had arrived. The first policeman walked in and took note of where the axe had hit the door, tracing the mark with his fingers.

He stepped into the clinic and said in an annoyed voice, 'If you girls can't hack it out here, then maybe you shouldn't be here?'

Those words felt like a slap in the face.

From behind him came a second voice; his partner was an older, heavy-set policeman

'Heard you were in Yulara for the weekend?' the older policeman said in an equally annoyed voice. 'You never rang me?' My heart sank. I felt like I was going to vomit. This was not the first time

I had met this policeman. He had come by my house one day with his partner for a chat about someone they were concerned about. I had offered them a coffee and we all sat and chatted in the comfort of my home. At the end of that chat, as I walked them to the door, he turned to me and looked into my eyes with a look of longing and loneliness. His gaze had slowly dropped down and lingered over my breasts before moving to my waist. When he looked up and met my gaze again, I felt so uncomfortable. I didn't know where to look so I focussed on his discoloured teeth while he spoke. Years of smoking and coffee had stained them, and I felt so repulsed by him at that moment. How dare he make me feel like this in my own home? I focussed on his teeth as he said, 'You know, if you ever want to go to Yulara on your weekend off, we (the police) get free accommodation. Just let me know; I will come and join you.' He'd had a stupid grin on his face as he looked over me one more time, like I was a piece of meat. I hadn't known how to respond, as I was always polite and didn't want to offend. But I felt so uncomfortable right then that all I could say was, 'Sure, no worries, mate,' casually and non-committed. 'Have a good day, guys,' I had said as I watched them walk out. I had closed the door and locked it.

Now here he was in the clinic, questioning why I had gone to Yulara without letting him know. I diverted the conversation by showing them the axe and the spear that Gloria had brought to the clinic to hide. I explained that there were reports of Billy being down at the big tree on the other side of the community, threatening to hang himself with his belt.

Both policemen walked out of the clinic to go and try to find Billy.

It felt like they had been gone for hours, but it was realistically just 30 minutes before Billy entered the clinic. He walked behind one of the policemen, who was holding an iced coffee in his hand. Billy walked up to me. In the presence of both policemen, he hung his head, not daring to look at me, as if he were ashamed. I tensely waited to see what he would do or say. One of the policemen prompted him: 'Billy has something he wants to say to you.'

He indicated to Billy that it was his turn to speak. Billy had a sandwich in his hand, a little less menacing since the last time he'd been here. They must have been at the store, because the other policeman was drinking a can of Coke. There was a long pause, as if Billy was thinking hard about what it was he should say. He lifted his head in silence and paused.

'Palya?' he said softly, looking up at me ever so briefly before looking down at the ground again.

That was it? One word. Palya. I was in disbelief, but then this was their culture, and just when you think that you understand, you realise how far apart our two worlds really are.

'Palya,' I replied, acknowledging him. With that one little word, it was as if the events of the day had all been erased. We were on good terms again, as if nothing had happened.

After I responded, he turned and glanced at the police, as if to say, 'See, we're good, there's no problem here.'

This prompted the policeman to speak. 'Billy said he was hungry and that is why he did it. We have given him a sandwich, so all is good. Isn't it, Billy? Now, you promised that if we got you the sandwich, you would have your needle.'

I prepared the injection and Billy sat there calmly, but I was still cautious. The police watched. I sensed they were impatient, so I hurried and gave Billy his antipsychotic injection.

After that was done, the other policeman turned to look at me. 'Look, in all honesty, the axe didn't touch you, so it isn't assault. We can probably get him for the damages to the door and floor.' His tone was matter of fact. I was in shock. I didn't know what to say or to think. I looked at Billy eating his sandwich. He had been rewarded for his bad behaviour.

With that, both the policeman and Billy left the clinic. I walked them out and locked the cage again. I stood there, staring out the window. I was locked in the clinic again, feeling abandoned. I felt let down. I knew I was free to leave, but my legs still felt weak. Right then, I just gave up on what needed to be done in the clinic. Suddenly it didn't matter. Nothing mattered.

Cut a Long Story Short

The following Friday, tears began to stream down my face as the mail plane took off from Pipalyatjara. I couldn't control them, so I tried to hide my face against the window so no one would see. There were three of us and the pilot on the flight to Alice Springs.

The Aboriginal lady sitting next to me reached out and touched my shoulder in a nurturing fashion acknowledging my pain. She said, 'Munta Kunga.' I stared out the window, unable to see through the tears as I tried to take in the view of Pipalyatjara from the air one last time. I felt broken and defeated.

I mourned the loss of seeing my favourite place again in all its glory, with wild flowers around the big red rock where I so often walked with the Aboriginal women. They had shown me the old artwork.

I mourned the elder women who had taken me out to the sacred women camps, welcoming me to ceremonies, and the cups of tea we drank in the clinic as we exchanged stories.

I mourned not being able to help the people in this community any more. I knew that I would be replaced, but would that person care like I cared? Or would it be just a job for them?

I mourned the feeling of peace and knowing that though I would always be an outsider here, having grown up in a remote area with Indigenous people, I felt at home here in the remoteness and thrived working independently. I was proud of my resilience while working autonomously in such harsh conditions. It took one bad person to change my course and although I might never return, the beautiful people in the APY lands will always remain in my heart.

***

The names in this have been changed to protect the identity of all of the people mentioned, except for my own. The place names and events have remained the same.

Glossary:

APY lands: Anangu Pitjantjatjara Yankunytjatjara lands, an area spanning the top of South Australia with many small remote Aboriginal communities

Watarru: Located in the west of the APY lands at Mt. Lindsay

Yulara: A tourist area just outside of Uluru-Kata Tjuta National Park

Pipalyatjara: The westernmost community in the APY lands close to the Western Australian border.

Pitjantjatjara: A dialect spoken by the Aboriginal people in Central Australia

Owa: yes

Wiya: no

Palya: okay

Munta: sorry

Pampa: old woman

Kunga: sister

Troopy: troop carrier vehicle used by police and ambulance for off-road driving.

CHAPTER 14

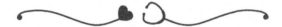

DR OLIVIA ONG

SPECIALIST PAIN MEDICINE AND
REHABILITATION PHYSICIAN

It should have been a great day. I got out of my car and walked through the hospital car park, the same path that I usually take to work. At the corner of my eye, I saw an old, worn-out 1980 Toyota reversing outwards from the disabled parking lot – and I didn't think much of it.

Everything happened so fast. The next thing I knew, I was thrown up in the sky and landed with a hard thud on the ground. I opened my eyes. Excruciating pain coursed through my lower back, and I could feel my body was twisted into an awkward position on the unforgiving concrete.

That car must have hit me.

But I'm still alive... Thank you, God, for protecting me and saving my life.

I mentally put on my rehab doctor's hat and did a head to toe inventory. My thinking was intact, so I must not have had a traumatic head injury. I started moving my right arm, followed by my left arm. I thought to myself that, given my arms were still functioning normally, I was not a quadriplegic. Then I realised I was not able to feel my legs. I panicked, thinking, *I hope I am not a paraplegic...* and then I realised that I was not able to move my legs, either. I suspected that I had a spinal cord injury; this was what the doctors called "spinal shock," where there is a loss of sensation accompanied by motor paralysis, with complete loss or weakening of all reflexes below the spinal cord injury. This phase lasts for a day. The neurons in various reflex arcs normally receive a basal level of excitatory stimulation from the brain. After a spinal cord injury, these cells lose this input and the neurons involved become hyperpolarised and less responsive to stimuli such as light, touch, temperature, and the sense where the joints of the body are.

Suddenly, a code blue was called in the hospital. "Code blue in the carpark. Code blue in the car park." A group of doctors rushed towards me. I recognised them. They were my peers, rehabilitation doctors that I was training with at the time. I realised that I WAS the code blue. The look of distress and concern on their faces was really apparent. My intuition told me that I was in it for the long haul; my life would never be the same again. I asked the senior rehab doctor, Dr Robin, whether I would be transferred to the main hospital where the car accident happened. After all, the hospital was where I had been working over the past few months. Dr Robin avoided my gaze and told me in a soft tone that the hospital was on bypass and that the Emergency Department was full, so I would be transferred to another tertiary hospital. I was very distressed and couldn't help but look at him angrily. I thought to myself: "How dare the hospital not take me! I am an employee there, after all!"

The paramedics came swiftly, and Dr Robin gave them a clinical handover before they put me on the stretcher for the ambulance. The siren was on and I was on my way to hospital – as a patient, not a doctor. I felt anxious that no one had called my husband to inform him that I'd been involved in a car accident and was on my way to hospital. I felt helpless lying on the stretcher, and I wished I had someone in the ambulance with me.

I was all alone.

The ambulance arrived at the major tertiary hospital and I was whisked away to the Emergency Department. I waited for a long time in the hospital bay, and my husband, John, finally was able to come in to see me. The orthopaedic doctor, Dr David, came and talked to me in a compassionate manner and organised for me to have a CT scan of my lower back. It felt weird being in the CT scan machine for the first time. The metal surface was cold, as was the radiology room where I was having the CT scan. The scan was over in less than 15 minutes. The porters whisked me back to the hospital bay in the Emergency Department, where John was waiting.

It felt like an eternity, but it was less than an hour before Dr David came in. He looked really sad. My heart sank, because deep down I knew things were not good at all. He informed me that I had a burst L2 vertebrae with L1 and L2 dislocation in my lower lumbar spine. *This can't be happening...* I thought. I was devastated. My life was ruined. My husband sat next to me, his face pale. He was sitting slumped and looked absolutely devastated when he heard the news. We looked at each other, speechless. Dr David also told me that I needed emergency spinal surgery that day. My husband signed the consent form.

As I was transported by the porters from the Emergency Department to the Operating Theatre, John walked alongside me, but as we reached the Operating Theatre, the door shut and I lost sight of him. I was so scared and distraught. We had never been apart, ever... What if we ended up being apart for the rest of my life, if I didn't make it out of the surgery alive?"

I looked around the Operating Theatre and closed my eyes; I was in so much emotional pain. I was so afraid I might die; as I knew, all too well, that extreme blood loss could be a complication of the surgery and lead to haemorrhagic shock.

Dr David came in with his boss, Dr Jane, the spinal trauma surgeon rostered on for that day. Both of them spoke to me gently about the details of the operation. I nodded and accepted my fate, then and there. I remember the anaesthetist putting in an intravenous line – and the next thing I knew, I woke up in the ward, disorientated. John was sitting in a chair nearby, tired and nodding on and off to sleep. Once again, I realised that I was alive and I thanked God for saving my life. Dr Jane came in after my surgery and explained to me what happened in a compassionate manner. I was very touched and grateful to her. I made the commitment to myself that once I learnt to walk again, I would physically walk up to her and shake her hand.

The first two weeks following my spinal surgery were hell on earth. I had so much acute pain in my lower back. The pain medications made me so drowsy, and I felt disorientated. Eventually, I improved clinically and was transferred to the rehabilitation hospital.

I spent four months in the rehabilitation ward learning how to live my life in my wheelchair. Everyday I had a therapy schedule to follow. Daily physiotherapy sessions, occupational therapy sessions, and medical nursing reviews. Physically, I had to learn to navigate the ward and the hospital in a wheelchair. Functionally, I learnt to use a slide board to transfer from bed to wheelchair and back. I looked around at the sad faces around me: people like me with spinal cord injuries, chained to our wheelchairs. I had to learn to do my bowel and bladder management from the specialist spinal nurses. I had lost all my dignity.

Friends stopped visiting me, as they were afraid to face an Olivia different to the one they used to know. Life stood still for me while I suffered, whereas my fellow medical peers moved on with their lives. Both John and I were suffering together. It was such a traumatic experience being a patient and not a doctor. I had lost all hope. My logical brain told me that, given the extent of the damage inflicted to my spinal cord, there was a slim chance that I would walk again.

One day, two months into my inpatient rehabilitation stay, I was eating lunch in the dining room of the rehabilitation hospital with a fellow spinal cord injured patient, Gerry. We were talking about our movie dates with our partners over the weekend as a trial run for community access in our wheelchairs. Suddenly, another fellow spinal cord injured patient, Rick, came into the dining room excitedly.

I asked Rick, "What's happening? You look really excited!"

Rick was talking really excitedly. "Have you heard of Project Walk, Olivia?"

I shook my head.

Rick went on to explain what Project Walk was all about. It was a rehabilitation centre in San Diego, California, that specifically helps people with spinal cord injuries to walk again. I was excited when I heard this. My intuition told me to pack my bags and head to Project Walk right away. However, that same night, I chose to ignore my intuition, and I ignored her for a very long time – 12 months in fact. But I never gave up my hope to walk again.

During my hospital stay, I went through the stages of grief every day. This included being in denial by pretending that the accident never happened to me and that it was just a bad dream. I went through anger, where I would be angry at God for letting such an accident happen to me. I went through sadness, where I daily for the loss of the use of my legs. I bargained with God – if I could walk again, I would help people in my plight walk again. I finally accepted that the accident had happened for a reason, that I did have faith in God, and that He would help me walk again.

John suffered, too. He became my caregiver and had to give up his full-time job to care for me. My spinal cord injury tested our marriage. My greatest regret was that I channelled my unhelpful, difficult emotions and feelings towards him during this time, and this was very unfair to him. Both of us were trying to manage our own suffering with whatever resources we had. He stayed by my side during this time and loved me unconditionally.

I was discharged from hospital in early 2009, after which John and I stayed at a supported accommodation while our house was renovated for modifications for my wheelchair. I had made some progress in my recovery; my left leg was functional, but my right leg remained very paralysed. I needed a Knee Above Foot Orthosis (KAFO) to fully support my right knee and right ankle in a fixed position, so that I could mobilise short distances using forearm crutches. I started working with a community physiotherapist on relearning to walk with the KAFO. At the end of 2009, a stance phase KAFO was fabricated for me by my orthotist to use functionally. Around early 2010, my physiotherapist told me that there was nothing else he could do for me, which made me feel so disappointed in him. I was ready to work extremely hard to walk again, yet everyone around me had given up on me. John and my family never gave up on me, though, so I continued to soldier on.

I started back at part-time work in late 2009, and this gave me a sense of purpose. It took a moment to get past the awkwardness of meeting my colleagues as the "new" me, in a wheelchair. Eventually, they came to realise that despite the wheelchair, I was still the same Olivia deep down. John and I started to readjust to life and to meet up with some friends, but this involved significant courage on my end. I was so scared of rejection from my friends.

In the end, my close friends accepted me for who I am, and they continued to support me no matter what.

My intuition is a very wise woman. She is very patient with me and never gave up on me. Each time I felt down in the dumps during those years pre-injury, and when I felt confined in the wheelchair, she was there to remind me to never give up hope, and that Project Walk was definitely the right step for me.

Have you ever heard your intuition telling you to follow your heart and pursue your dreams, only for logic to kick in, telling you that you aren't good enough? Not worthy enough, so you give up on your dream?

Intuition, which is also known as gut feelings, can give you a vibe that something is not quite right. Experienced doctors know when a patient's story just doesn't add up. Intuition helps us in complex medical decision making. Clinical evidence can only take us so far; the heart and gut must speak.

Us doctors also tend to ignore our intuition when listening to patients and during diagnosis and management of our patients. Instead, logic kicks in. When we suppress our intuition, our heart, which yearns to be a creator (be it writing, music, or art), is unable to speak.

I will never forget the moment I heard my intuition speak much more strongly than it had before. I remember this defining moment so clearly. I was lying on the bed alone at night, wondering what my life would be like without the use of my legs, and whether I would be a doctor again. Whether my husband would love me again, whether I would have children. Then, my inner knowing told me to pack my bags and leave for San Diego to attend the Project Walk Recovery Center. A centre to help people with spinal cord injuries walk again.

I did just that. I told my boss that I would be away from work for two years to focus on my rehabilitation. He was compassionate and told me to strive for my dreams to walk again.

In March 2010, the day before our flight to San Diego, I packed my bags, full of hope and promise. Every fibre of my being told me it was a heart-centred decision.

My recovery at Project Walk involved hours of physical therapy and acupuncture. My supportive husband accompanied me to San Diego and was there by my side at every moment.

We made beautiful memories in San Diego, met many friends, and travelled around the USA and Canada while I was still in a wheelchair. We went to Las Vegas on the 4th of July, to Universal Studios in Burbank, California, and to Disneyland in Anaheim on the weekends. Thankfully, the USA is extremely wheelchair accessible and so I was able to get around the cities relatively easily. The most memorable trip was to New York City; it truly became my most favourite city in the world. It was really tough doing intensive physical therapy day in, day out, but the friendships that I made remain as untouchable, beautiful memories that will last a lifetime.

On a typical fall day in Carlsbad, California, in the Project Walk gym, I was training with my lead trainer, Michelle. She was holding my arms as I started walking around unassisted and said, "I am going to let go of you, Olivia."

I blinked at Michelle and said: "You gotta be kidding, right? What if I fall down and hit my head? What if I fall down and break my hip, leg, etc.?" As a doctor, I went straight to worst-case scenarios.

Michelle just smiled at me and said, "Trust me, you got this."

I took my first step unassisted cautiously, then the next step and the next step. Before I knew it, I was walking around the gym on my own two feet, finally able to leave footprints on the grounds of the gym. What an awesome feeling!

"The doctor is back in the house. I can walk again." I beamed at Michelle. This was my defining moment, nearly two long, agonising years after my accident, I was able to walk again. I looked at Michelle and smiled the biggest smile in the world. What had just happened?

Michelle had just let go of my hands, and I walked out of the wheelchair, all on my own – strong, defiant, resilient, fighter.

When I returned to Melbourne, Australia, in 2012, I resumed my training as a registrar in Rehabilitation Medicine. I started with part-time work followed by full-time work.

I really love how funny life can turn out to be. I met Dr Jane one day when she was giving the rehabilitation medicine registrars a lecture on Spinal Surgery. When the lecture ended, I walked up to Dr Jane. She looked at me and initially did not seem to recognise me. I spoke to her and asked, "Remember me, Dr Jane? I was that registrar you operated on five years ago?" It finally registered to her who I was and we shook hands. It was such an emotional moment.

"You are walking now?" she exclaimed. "That's amazing!"

"Yes," I said with a smile. "I went to Project Walk San Diego and learnt to walk again, and it's been two years now."

When I returned to Melbourne to resume my work as a doctor, my clinical practice changed because of my experiences with spinal cord injury. I was more empathetic towards my patients and could understand where they were coming from, listening to them intuitively. I was starting to get into the "heart-centredness" of medicine.

Over the next eight years, I went on to build up a successful private practice in rehabilitation and pain medicine as a dual-trained rehabilitation medicine and pain physician. I went on to have two beautiful children: Joseph, who is now five years old, and Jacqueline, who is now ten months old. I am leading a heart-centered life that I truly deserve. I have implemented intuition in my role as a doctor and as a mum to two children. I am a lot kinder to myself, more mindfully aware of my difficult emotions and thoughts, especially by just observing them, with no judgement or self-criticism. All of this has helped me to become a better doctor. Because I am so in tune with my intuition, I can intuitively listen to my patients, and they feel more supported. In essence, I felt wholeheartedly what the heart of medicine is all about.

I knew that my life was destined for something greater. The accident was the beginning of a transformative journey for me. My life would never going to be the same again. I have learned to always rely on my intuition in any minor and major decisions in my life.

I took the next level of direction of being a holistic pain physician, incorporating self-compassion and creative development practice into my clinical work, which solidified my heart in medicine. I empower my patients with knowledge and medical and holistic pain management treatments to manage their chronic pain, neurological disabilities, and/or rehabilitation so they can live fulfilling lives.

My vision for 2021 is to encourage doctors to cultivate self-compassion and a creative development practice that helps them feel that their heart is rightly placed in the field of medicine.

Ultimately, my global mission is to help fellow doctors suffering from emotional and physical burnout to uncover the benefits of intuitive techniques, for not just for themselves, but their patients, too.

CHAPTER 15

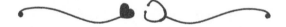

DR SIMONE WATKINS

DOCTORAL STUDENT, PAEDIATRIC ADVANCED TRAINEE AND PROFESSIONAL TEACHING FELLOW

Dear 19-year-old self,

You are more than just a nice, hard-working brown girl.
You can be more than what others say you should be.
You can redefine that box.

There is a lot to explain on this day, when you are about to embark on the journey to becoming a medicine woman. You are about to be face-to-face with the enduring, provocative, and dominating societal view that doctors are white males. But instead of trying, with difficulty, to fit this mould, you can break out of this ridiculous proverbial box.

I'm writing to you now because you start medical school after the summer, and it is a significant milestone in shaping who you will become. I know this because I am you. I am 33-year-old Simone, writing to you from the future. I write to you lovingly, with not only tender warnings but also inspiration to comfort you. I see you driving around town with the top down in the cream beetle, carefree and full-spirited with your friends, full of hope and expectation about what the future will hold.

But please know, although your life in 2021 will not look how you expected, trust me – you will become so much more than you realise. This letter calls on you to keep in mind that life is a summation of your choices, so choose wisely. You don't have to be who people want or expect you to be. You can just be uniquely you. You can carve out your own beautiful, imperfectly messy, and at times unexpected life path.

First off: Congratulations.

I know you feel elated to have made it into medical school. What a crucial milestone in determining what the future holds for you. All of the hard work in that first year of university has paid off, and you can stop competing with peers and finally make life-long friends and allies. Being accepted into medical school is such a massive achievement, considering how, at the age of 13, you still fainted at the sight of blood and required your friends to "doctor" your stubbed toe.

I know how grateful you feel, especially on this day of outstanding achievement, for what your parents sacrificed and gave for you to be where you are today. On reflecting, your parents are such an inspiration to you and will continue to be throughout your career as a doctor. Your legacy continues to be built on their history: Your mother, growing up with a single parent in poverty in a small-town north of Auckland, who became a successful businesswoman; and your father, immigrating to Auckland at the age of 12 from Samoa, who became a successful director of an accounting firm. The critical path they shaped has allowed you to be where you are today. You know they worked up society's hierarchical social ladder for you and your two siblings. For you to be an influence, they put you through private school, and I remember how you gritted your teeth and stubbornly didn't want them to pay for your university. You shut the door of your room and studied extremely hard to enable you to be awarded a full university scholarship, relieving them of that cost.

Your innate drive, to almost prove something for your parents' sake, is an overall great trait. But it does have a dark side, so watch out. Continued striving can be tiring in itself. You don't need to strive and succeed to be enough. You were born enough.

You are smart.

You are so incredibly intelligent. You may not project this intelligence at all times, but I hope you know it is in you. Remember when you started school and you didn't realise, but you were in a mixed class with children a year older than you? This meant you learned everything a year ahead, and it came naturally to you. Don't worry about people who talk to you and assume you couldn't have gotten A's in your exam last year. In the upcoming years, you will hear many sentiments such as "We were so surprised you could XYZ!" Don't underestimate or undervalue yourself because of these off-hand comments. People will continue to assume, and you can't change how others react and respond to you, but you can change your internal dialogue and reaction to people.

Please, don't worry about others. Theodore Roosevelt said *"comparison is the thief of joy"* for a reason. Just feel content with what brain you have been given. Although – *spoiler alert* – your brain probably does lead to a future relationship breakup when your perceived lack of studying for your most critical medical school exams causes a certain boy to become frustrated. Don't worry. You graduate with distinction from the top tier of your medical school graduate class without him. Get out of fight mode, because there is nothing you have to prove.

In saying this, please keep your charmingly absent-minded "blonde" moments (in fact, for a brief period in 2020/21, you will bleach your hair blonde and blame your blonde behaviours on your hair colour!). You and your high school friends will still look back on the unforgettable day where you were pretty ditzy indeed. I'm sure you recall when you and your friends were all in the kitchen. You, leaning on the kitchen bench, while your friend (who happens to be blonde), who has known you since intermediate school, pours you a Coca-Cola (coke) into a glass alongside everyone else's glasses. You slowly pick up the glass, stare at it intensely, and genuinely ask, "Is this blue coke in my glass?!?" to which your friends all just stare blankly at you with incredulous looks on their faces. After a reasonably awkward pause, your friend exclaims that the drinking glass is coloured blue and the Coke is, in fact, just regular, plain Coke. Wow. What a day. It continues to bring smiles to us all when we recall the hilarity of that moment. Leading to your friends' favourite joke: "...and you're a doctor?!?"

Your job does not define you.

Remember in the future, only five years away, that being a doctor does not define you.

I know you began this journey to become a doctor because of a higher purpose and calling. Your job is your vocation, and of course, it will be a part of your life and who you are. But, in fact, at the time of writing, you are taking time out from your clinical job. So please, love your job, but know that your job is not your everything.

There are dangers in being defined by a job. It is an unstable footing. Your job, as you learn, can be taken away at any moment, by sickness or other uncontrollable factors. You are yet to learn about things that you cannot control – but do not fear the loss of control. There will be freedom when you uncouple your self-image and self-esteem from your vocation. You indeed are a compassionate doctor, but being a doctor also means always giving of yourself. Be careful. If you keep giving them pieces of yourself, you will not have anything left.

You can (and will) be defined by so much more than your vocation – you are caring, loving, loyal, and hold fast to your values. You stand strong, no matter the undercurrents around you. A beautiful indigenous Māori proverb also speaks of this: "*Kia Kaha, Kia Maia, Kia Manawanui,*" which translates to "Be strong, be brave, be steadfast." Hold fast to these values, and you will stand in integrity. Being true to yourself is one of the most important life principles.

Being a doctor is hard some days, but it's worth it for the good days.

You are about to enter into another life chapter after medical school – the junior doctor world. Your university sets you up well academically and practically for the world of practicing medicine. But what they cannot teach you, you learn the hard way, for how can one teach you how to face human fragility and vulnerability, death and dying, difficult conversations, work politics, and life-or-death decisions?

To point out the obvious, you also are a bubbly, somewhat naïve, 24-year-old afakasi Samoan girl when you begin your journey as a doctor. There will be practically no one who looks like you where you try to go – the majority of leaders and professors are European (white) and male. But that is okay. You will be okay. You have a unique stance, viewpoint, and worldview. You don't have to copy others to be accepted or successful.

Other peoples' comments do not help you to feel motivated to be all you can be. There will be many critical commentaries and observations of your life and how you should live it. For example, "You are too nice to be a surgeon." There will even be requests and recommendations, but take heart: You do not need to listen to everyone all the time – just live and speak your own truths. Overcome your fear and step into your dreams for your own good. The need to comply with others' ideas for your acceptance is not necessary. Neither is overworking to prove yourself. You can do what you want. You can be who you like. Don't let others stop you.

The choice of who you will be in your career is difficult. The options seem endless. After a few years of circling and chasing your tail regarding choosing a specialty career path, you will begin your training as a registrar in your preferred specialty. I will not reveal that to you now, because that is a journey you will need to go on. Just know your specialty makes you smile every day, and it gives you so much job satisfaction. There is so much joy in knowing you are helping to make people well again. Follow your passion, your skills, and your joy, and it will all make sense.

You marry and find unconditional love.

To further my last point, somebody you work with in hospital will tell you, "No one will want to date you because you are too intimidating, you are gorgeous and intelligent, men can't handle that." But you are not a gold ring in a pig's snout. You have an extremely high moral character and are worthy of love. Your outward appearance has nothing to do with the innermost parts of your authentic being. And that list of attributes you hope to find in a husband that you have concocted – please throw that away! Higher forces know that what you need is not what you want.

You find a type B life partner to match your type A. You need this – you work in a high tension, high stress, fast-paced workplace called the public hospital. You also start at the bottom of the hospital system's perpetual hierarchical culture, which has its own layers of difficulty. Your husband will teach you how to navigate that place by effectively communicating and managing people. He hates being late places, though, so now would be a good time for you to buy a watch and practice being more punctual.

The love of your life is like love at first sight for you (maybe not as much for him), and he will joke that you are annoying. Nonetheless, he is a needed constant in your life. He will never give up on you and loves you so authentically for who you are. It is overwhelming sometimes. He will see your dark days, crazy moments, achievements, and life milestones, but throughout it all he will always remain steadfast and your number one supporter. True love with no conditions is hard to find, but you find this rarity when you least expect it, and a whirlwind of adventure starts from there – so be expectant and excited.

You will have a family.

You have heard, "Don't become a doctor, because then you won't be able to be a mother," and you will listen to "Don't get pregnant before your specialist written exam." Luckily, you are stubborn and go your own way anyway. This does mean you cannot sit your specialist written exam when you initially planned because you'll be passing a different kind of life milestone, becoming a parent.

Right now, time may seem like a non-changing constant where each day and night is the same length. Yet, as a parent, this is not the case – time somehow warps itself, and days seem to go on forever while weeks pass by quickly. And then, just like that, you stop and realise that the status of your life influences your sense of time at that moment. Appreciating time is a privilege. Being a mother is a privilege. Being a doctor who is now a parent is a privilege.

However, although being a mother is something of importance to you, actually becoming a mother will not be an easy journey. So, make your career how you want, and it will work out. You will have to quit the rat race and walk off the conveyor belt of career-ship producing specialist doctors and off-road your journey. Still, this road is much more fun, and it will take you places you never thought you would go.

Your children will teach you so much. Some unexpected challenges arise, but instead of living in a life of "what could be" or "what should be" or "but why," you decide to intentionally say that your children are as they are for a purpose. As a mother, you will love them unconditionally. This means accepting them as they are and encouraging them to grow and be the best person they can be. Society may set its own "normal," but striving to be this impractical image is fruitless when you and your future children were born to be different. To stand out. Besides, to have a unique platform to speak your truth is such a gift.

Having a child that is different from expected means life will have more complications. There are some things you cannot plan for. Consequently, you will sacrifice for love. You will lay down your own needs and plans to fulfil your most important calling – being a mother.

Fortunately, you never regret it or feel bitter because gratitude brings contentment. Your children can propel you into a new direction, where your career focuses on promoting social justice, inclusion, and fair treatment for all. All humans have the innate capacity to give and receive love, and all are deserving of this love and respect.

Stay kind, even when others are not.

The real world out there can be harsh. Cynicism is present in epidemic proportions. And you, as a naïve, innocent soul, can be misinterpreted. This means that there will be people who will question your motives – but that will say more about them than you. Stay genuine.

A charge nurse will ask, "Why did you get me this coffee? Are you trying to persuade me to give you a good review?" A male consultant will ask, "Why did you bake this cake? Are you trying to butter us up? When I baked a cake, all the nurses were so impressed!" A work colleague will tell you, "It doesn't matter what you do because you are so replaceable."

However, consider this: Kindness and love transcend language and culture. Genuineness is in your eyes. There will be a time when you step up into a role that is well beyond your experience and level of training, but you will bring genuineness, and it will be apparent to others around you. Although some will misinterpret, misunderstand, and be confused by you, just continue to be yourself. When you feel like you're stepping up, with big shoes to fill, don't try to replicate how others work or succeed because it will not translate. You only need to be yourself, with your daft jokes and big smile. You will continue to see good in others, defend others, speak well of people, and encourage all around you. Kindness is a fundamental part of you.

Practice self-love.

Others need kindness because you don't know what they are going through or have been through. But **you** need kindness because others don't see what you have gone through. Don't forget to be kind to yourself. A staunch appearance when you're as fragile as glass will not fool everyone. You cannot be everything, to all people, all of the time. It is not possible. So just breathe, be compassionate to yourself, and let your emotional love-tank be completely full so you have the capacity to overflow to others. In other words, you do not need to be perfect.

New Zealand, although a small country of five million people, is known for tall poppy syndrome. I believe tall poppy syndrome comes from peoples' insecurity and fear. So, when you feel targeted by others, don't focus on their cut-downs or confrontations. New Zealand has a culture of wanting everyone to be on one level, so being successful or standing out in a crowd can be intimidating to some. Know who your trusted people are and listen to them. Don't just listen to everyone and take everyone's comments to heart. That leads to you feeling like you need to be someone different to be liked and accepted. This should not and will not be the case when you love and accept yourself for who you are. What is more, the insightful eye of another will identify your potential. Being stretched almost continually to grow exponentially as a trainee and graduate doctor can be painful. Reaching for your potential is not always comfortable, but the rewards are great.

Accepting yourself and celebrating your wins in life is one thing, but taking the knocks along the way and getting back up is hard. You will get knocked down and feel burnt out, but know that it's okay not to be okay. It is not a weakness to ask for help or to be vulnerable to those you trust. It is not personal when difficulties arise. To illustrate, you will fail in the future, but that will work out for the best. Your character needs to grow and be refined. It will take failure to learn that to lose does not mean you are a loser. You can't attribute your character to your outcomes or who you are to your losses. Every one of the greats in history has failed, got it wrong, or lost things in life. Because that is life. I know you have met mainly success in your journey to date, but now (for your future self), I appreciate that I am where I am because those who went before me believed in me, helped me, encouraged me, and gave me opportunities to thrive and grow.

You have inspirational mentors and supervisors in your future. Remember them and thank them. It is an honour to walk behind these great people and stumble but have a steady hand to help you rise again. Everyone can break. But when you are ready, you will realise there are things you can do that you didn't believe you could. You have a hidden reservoir of strength within you.

Sometimes, you have to be broken down to be built up stronger with added reinforcements. In construction, *strengthening* is the process of **upgrading** a structural building system in order to increase its capacity and performance when carrying additional loads. Perhaps at times you look at the load you feel you carry and it pushes the limits of your current capacity. Maybe deeper foundations needed to be laid in order to increase your influence. You will hear a song in the future with which you will strongly connect, titled "Dismantle, Repair," by the band Anberlin. Sometimes a dismantle may be required before repair. We cannot become stronger without dismantling habits, thoughts, and behaviours that are not helpful in aligning us with our bigger purpose in life. In a classic Kiwi DIY ("do it yourself") rebuild, the "demo" stage is when you demolish or take down in order to leave space to rebuild. For you, this will be rebuilding more strength, more courage, more boldness, more perseverance, and more resilience.

Although at times you may not feel worthy or good enough, please remember that I know the truth about your future. Do not be fearful. You will rebuild that misguided dialogue and be redirected through life's difficult circumstances. There will be **beauty out of the ashes** when you emerge with increased capacity and strength.

It is not on the mountaintop that we necessarily find ourselves or who our people are – it's in the desert or the valley. During your time of rebuilding yourself, you write a poem about the whole experience:

In the wilderness, we develop
Developing strength and courage
Courage to face ourselves
Our own shortcomings
And our own strengths
Courage to face the world
The crazy, complex, and at times cruel world
But within the craze lies beauty, resilience, character
And if you wait patiently enough – joy.

Do you agree, maybe it is a powerful word?
A word of things that could be
When would be or should be's
Become too much to bear
Maybe, allows a breath of fresh air
The space to begin to realign and renew
To create and just wait, without having to do
Healing takes time and space
But that is okay, we can go at our own pace.

Sometimes a pause isn't as bad as it seems
We pause and wait for hope
There is more we can do than just cope
Perhaps room for us now will lead us to find
All we needed from each other was to be kind
As you were to all the others while neglecting
Your own thoughts and feelings
You needed to try to keep your sanity
Being face to face with gritty humanity.

Slowly you start to give out again
You give over your life instead of just hold
So stand up, shout, it is time to be bold
About what you need and like and hold dear
Because there is no movement when there is just fear
Be brave, my friend, and you might find
There is space to be free of the bind
To find a purpose with joy overflow
I believe it will mean more than you know.

Your circumstances do not define you.

For the phoenix rising from the ashes... is you.

You have a voice. And you will use it.

A high school teacher spoke over you and said to your parents, "Simone isn't very good at writing; don't expect her to get excellences or good grades in English this year." Nevertheless, you will show them that anything is possible. The impossible for you now can become possible with hard work, perseverance, and a resilient spirit. Don't disqualify yourself before you even start. If you want to say something strongly enough, your passion will come through.

I know you don't think this could be true, but future you is currently committed to writing a 100,000-word thesis. You will avoid research like it is the plague reincarnate, but your journey to your thesis is not a straight line. Within your future thesis, you plan to practically help your Samoan people. It is your heritage; it is a part of who you are. You will do this by investigating if there are any contributing factors to ethnic inequalities in health outcomes (I know, so nerdy, right?). But how astonishing that you are able to practically make your written teenage goals and dreams come true.

Finally, I hope this letter becomes embedded in your heart – for your life matters. Take heed of my warnings and allow yourself to flourish.

Go forth and conquer, 19-year-old Simone.

Love,

Your future self (33-year-old you)

xx

"Live a life worthy of the calling you have received."

CHAPTER 16

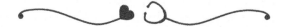

REBECCA LANG
NATUROPATH & NUTRITIONIST

"Mum, Mum, look! Cheetah's in the middle of the road!" screamed my son.

We had just driven home to Bargara on the coast of Bundaberg, Queensland, from Noosa, in torrential rain. I could barely see in front of me. As we arrived on the main road where we lived, there was a power pole down, blocking the street and the entrance to our driveway. There were broken tree branches and debris from houses scattered all along the road. There were birds and what sounded like a possum screeching the sounds of death. The air was humid and the smell of salt and seaweed off the ocean was strong. The police suddenly appeared, sirens blaring, and yelled at us to go home and not be out on the road. I tried to tell them that this was our home, but they couldn't hear me amongst the billowing wind and pouring rain. They just blocked the road and signalled for me to turn around. It was raining outside, but I started to sweat in panic. My son looked at me with wide, scared eyes. What had happened to our quiet, safe beachside town?

My friend's house was across the street from ours, so we parked in her driveway. She wasn't home, but I didn't know what else to do, so I broke into her house through an unlocked window. My son and I sat inside her lounge, at her front window, staring

161

in shock at our home. All the fences were down, tree branches everywhere, and our beloved, 13-year-old dog, confused and lost in the middle of the road.

It was mid-afternoon 27 January, 2013. The power was out, and as I sat with my 12-year-old son, we saw that the roof of the house next to ours was off, as was the one next to that. Ours appeared to still be on, but we couldn't see the back of the house. There was debris all over the road and streets. Our only contact with what was happening was Facebook on my phone, where we saw that a tornado had gone through our little town only moments prior to our return from Noosa. There was still a risk of further tornados, with water spouts still appearing at the coast.

After a few hours of trying to be patient, I finally ran over to our home in the rain. I couldn't wait a moment longer before ensuring our pets were safe, and all I could think about in the chaos was to wonder where I had put the photo albums. I am known in my family as the 'keeper of old things' so I had been given the duty of looking after precious family memorabilia. Fortunately, I found our two cats were safely inside, hiding under the bed. The house was dry, but the roof was damaged on one side of my bedroom and over the main bathroom. The house, horseshoe-shaped, meant that the back of the house had some damage but the front of the house was okay. I breathed a sigh of relief once I had ensured that all of the precious family items were safe and moved them and our passports into my old wooden glory box.

The backyard looked like a scene from *Jumanji*. All the outdoor furniture and plants were upside down and strewn across the expanse of green lawn. My neighbour had a massive Moreton Bay fig tree in her backyard – and now every branch of that tree was either in my backyard and on my roof. Birds and bats and other creatures lay amongst the branches, crushed to death. The smell of salt and death was strong. The garage door was bent open, its roof damaged. Rain poured into the shed. I wondered if there were any precious items in there to worry about, but then realised there wasn't any chance of getting over the debris to the shed and so decided to not even worry about it.

My naturopathic clinic, located at the front of the house, had escaped most of the damage. My files were all still paper files at this stage, and so I was grateful to see everything safe and dry in this area – and resolved to get everything online in the near future!

By 6pm, the rain started to ease up, and we went over to see our neighbours. Their roofs were off, but some of them had gathered and for a few drinks. I couldn't understand why. I felt we needed to start packing their belongings immediately, but they felt hopeless, to say nothing of being overwhelmed by the loss of their roofs. Feeling the need to help, I went into my neighbour's son's room and packed his Xbox, new school uniforms, books, and clothes. I started to carry things to my house. I offered storage to my other neighbours but they were too overwhelmed and politely declined. I packed as much as I could for them, not stopping until midnight. By then, the rain had stopped and I guess they thought it might be okay.

As I got into bed, heavy rain started up again and went all night. I knew what was left in their homes would now be damaged.

Over the next five days, we had no power. I went out to my Jumanji backyard, stepping over dead animals, and found the gas stove and gas bottle in the wet shed. We used the gas stove for cooking, while an esky with ice saved what food we could. The rain eventually eased, but it was summer in Queensland and so the humidity was unbearable.

While we were in survival mode, Bundaberg – the local town, 25 minutes away – had flooded. The rivers rose with the heavy rain; houses were flooded, and the whole town became a disaster zone. We also learnt there had been five tornadoes in the surrounding coastal suburbs. I continued to help neighbours and friends as much as I could, knowing that I was one of the lucky ones. I was so exhausted one night that I just sat on the floor in the shower. But I felt guilty, that I should still be out there helping others.

Many people, including myself, pushed themselves so hard during this time, helping with the clean-up. We saw each other at the shops or on the streets and no words were needed. People were broken and exhausted. It would just be a nod of the head, a listless stare into the dark circles surrounding our eyes. There was no point in wasting time wearing makeup or dressing up nice. Every moment was spent helping others.

In Bundaberg, there was a massive clean-up to-do for houses and businesses. Washing machines and all sorts of debris kept showing up in the ocean and in the river. People volunteered to clean up flooded areas, walking through and working in contaminated flood water. Many people had issues with insurance companies refusing to cover their homes. Some people didn't have insurance. Families and friends and the community as a whole opened their homes to those in need, many taking in whole families for months on end. The catteries and pet hotels were overbooked; rental properties that hadn't been damaged were in high demand as people became homeless. Many people had lost their businesses and their jobs.

Prior to the natural disaster, I had been running my naturopathic clinic from home six days a week. I was already burnt out. I thought that the clinic would be quiet. But instead, it was busier than ever. People needed my help. The doctors' surgeries were also booked out. People were waiting weeks for an appointment. Many people were suffering from anxiety, depression, post-traumatic stress, and insomnia, as well as a whole range of physical symptoms. Working in the floodwaters put a lot of people's health at risk, as any type of open wound can become very infected, and the bacteria spread quickly. Many people also had skin conditions and respiratory illnesses, and a large number of people also developed a range of viral symptoms that had no medical diagnosis. Mould was growing quickly in houses as well, causing a range of health issues.

While I was working six days a week, with back-to-back clients, I still had tarps on the back of my house over the bedrooms and bathrooms. I was barely sleeping at all; any small amount of wind or rain put me in a state of panic and my adrenaline would kick in. Due to the unique horseshoe shape of my house, the insurance assessors were unsure what to do with it, so in the meantime I just had to survive with a temporary and partial roof over my bedroom and the back of the house.

As the weeks went on, I could not say no to anyone in need. I thought about having a Saturday off to rest, but people would ring up needing my help, and I couldn't turn them away. These people had gone through much more than me. My clients were still going to the doctor when they could get in, but we were using herbs and nutrients to support their immune systems, mental health, and symptoms. Many people also just needed emotional, mental, and spiritual support.

The two houses next to me were classed as complete write-offs by the insurance companies, and their owners were now in temporary housing.

It wasn't until March that my insurance company finally worked out what to do with my roof. To keep to council regulations, they had no choice but to replace the whole roof and some of the walls. Which would also mean repainting the house. So I was told we would have to move out, and that it could take three to four months to complete all the repairs due to the demand on the local building industry. The only problem was that by this stage, there was no housing available in the town and nowhere to look after our dog and two cats. Between my insomnia from not having a proper roof over my bedroom and a history of anxiety, I worked hard to keep my mind positive.

I continued consulting every day except Sunday, while I worried about what to do and where to go. I was at the stage with my busy clinic that my one-hour lunch break meant that I would be lucky to have five minutes to quickly eat something. I often ran late, giving as much as I could to help those in need.

I dragged out my decision as long as possible, until the insurance company said I had to make a decision, and could I stay with my family who were in Perth? On the other side of the country. With no real other options available, the decision was made, and I started the process of packing up 12 years of belongings and held $1 garage sales to reduce the packing. Why do we accumulate so much?

Meanwhile, I continued to consult; the clinic was the very last thing I packed. I booked my clients in for phone and video consultations for their next appointments. A truck turned up and collected all my boxes and some minimal furniture. My herbs, natural medicines, and client files were the last items to be packed. I consulted right up until the day before the truck arrived. The next day, I woke up with the worst flu I had ever had. I was sleeping on an air mattress and could barely get out of bed. All my natural remedies were packed.

The next night, I had some cold and flu tablets, knowing I had to start the drive across Australia the next morning. Unfortunately, I had an allergic reaction to them which restricted my breathing. I spent the next few days in bed. The insurance company rang, clients were ringing, and I finally got the strength to get in the car with my son and my dog and start the long drive across Australia.

After four days of driving, we finally arrived in Perth. I started to get better, but only two weeks later, I contracted another flu. This one was worse than the previous one. My herbs and natural medicines were locked in a storage holding facility, and so I just suffered through it, too exhausted to even think about accessing anything else.

Two weeks later, I started phone and video consulting for my Queensland clients. I finally was able to access my files and medicines from the storage unit. I dosed myself up and knew it was time to start helping others again. It seemed to work well, as my clients felt they were still getting the support they needed. I spent my evenings bubble-wrapping their products and getting them ready to post across Australia. At that time, there was no patient direct ordering, which would have made my life so much easier. I spent many hours lining up at the post office with ten or more packages. I also had many new clients booking in with me from Queensland. They were referred by family or friends, and even though I was on the other side of the country, they needed my help. Perth people started booking appointments, too.

I visited my home town in Queensland every two or so months and worked from a hotel. I saw over 50 clients in four or five days and then was back on a plane to Perth. My son was in school in Perth, and I couldn't be away from him for long. As my clients came in and referred others, I was shocked at how many people were sick. The floods had left unknown diseases. The doctors' surgeries were now booked a month or more ahead, as there seemed to be so many viruses around. I had left my home in April, and it wasn't until December that my house repairs were finished. It was never meant to take that long. The insurance company kept telling me it was to do with my unique house structure and that it had taken several engineers before they could decide what to do about it.

During this time in Perth, I did manage to have more downtime than in the previous few years. I was busy, but my consultations were 30 mins instead of the 60 minutes I had been doing in my clinic. Yet, I found myself feeling completely exhausted, and some days I struggled to get out of bed. At the very least, I started to need a nap at 2pm every day. Working from home, I had this option, and though I tried to fight it, by 2pm my eyes were closing and my body and mind went into shutdown.

I had seen this many times in my clients, particularly after the floods. I was going into adrenal burnout. I had been pushing myself for so long, putting myself last while I concentrated on helping others. I felt that if I had any energy in me, it should be given towards helping someone in need. But now I was the person in need.

I looked back and it all made sense. When I finally stopped to drive to Perth, my immune system went down. One of the first signs of adrenal burnout is a lowered immune system. Other signs included waking up tired, or crashing by 9am; you keep going and crash again after lunch; keep going and by 2pm you hit a wall. Dinner time is when people often crash again, and in early stages of adrenal burnout, the cortisol kicks in at night. Usually around 9pm. So while the rest of the world sleeps, you have more energy than you have had all day, which also results in disrupted sleep. And then you wake up in the morning to do it all over again. I was mindful that exhaustion can also bring on anxiety and depression. I had always experienced anxiety, but I had learned to manage it.

I improved my nutritional intake of food and cold-pressed juices, ensured I was getting some movement such as yoga, rested, and created my script of natural medicines, addressing any deficiencies and using herbs and nutrients to support my adrenal glands and cellular energy.

When I was finally able to move back to Queensland, there were further issues before I was able to move back into my home. Due to various circumstances, myself and my son found ourselves homeless for over six months, relying on friends and weekend stays and keeping our belongings in storage and basic items in the car. It was a very stressful time.

We were finally able to move into our home in July 2014. I then restarted my clinic from home. My energy had started to improve, and I was excited to be back in a position of really helping people. This time, though, I employed staff to support me. This took a lot of pressure off me, but instead of using this extra energy to look after myself, I took on mentoring for other naturopaths and students and before long I was booked out with an Internship

Program for naturopaths and nutritionists. The clinic was booked out as well, and I was back working six days a week.

After a couple of years, I was once again hit with fatigue and had to sneak a nap in on my lunch breaks. I had been struggling with insomnia – and cortisol kicking in at night – but now I could barely stay awake past 9pm. I moved next door to my home/clinic while I worked out what to do. This space next door gave me extra rest time. I would go there on my lunch breaks for a sleep before consulting in the afternoons. Meanwhile, I was dosing up on herbs and nutrients to support my adrenals and fatigue, but I knew deep inside that something had to change.

I decided to move my clinic to the CBD in my town, Bargara. I needed to have my home back. The perfect space became available, and while making this change, I also moved my hours to only consult Tuesdays, Wednesdays, and Thursdays. This gave me Mondays to prepare for the week and attend to other business obligations. Fridays were to rest and restore. I found the separation from my home really helped my energy levels as well.

I was feeling rested and rejuvenated, so I spontaneously opened a juice bar/vegan café next to my clinic: Of The Earth Juice Bar & Health Shop. I was really excited to be able to offer my clients and the community cold-pressed juices, dairy-free smoothies, organic coffee, and a three-day juice cleanse. Everything we made was gluten, dairy, and sugar free, and it was vegan and mostly raw. I knew from supporting my own body and nutrients that we needed easy access to healthier food.

What I didn't realise was that initially, it was going to take a lot of energy from me. I had staff, but I had to make sure things were done the way I had planned and that everything was not only nutritious but also looked amazing and tasted delicious.

The café was open from 6am to 5pm, seven days a week. What was I thinking? So here I was, getting there at 6am with a staff member and preparing juices, talking to people, doing dishes, and mopping floors before I went over to my clinic to consult. Weekends I would call in for an hour and end up there all day. It was a lot of fun to do something different and to make delicious, healthy food. However, I was also under a lot of financial stress with this new venture.

The juice bar had been open for about eight months when I attended a business retreat. It was when I stopped that I realised that once again I was exhausted. Except this time it was different. I could feel this darkness sitting right next to me. I turned and faced it and realised that I was about to be overtaken by depression. I felt the room closing in on me and everything seemed large. I couldn't breathe. I had always suffered with anxiety and some insomnia, but I had learnt to deal with these. Depression that was this dark and deep was something I had not experienced. The feeling of it being so close made me realise that when this overtakes you, it isn't just a matter of changing your way of thinking – it is beyond your control. I spent most of the retreat resting.

I went back home and decided to take a big step back from my juice bar. My staff knew what to do. From that day onwards, I have not mopped the floor, made juices, or done the dishes. I have realised that I don't need to do that anymore. I didn't go into the depression that was creeping up. I realised that if I didn't stop, then it was going to overtake me very quickly.

So, once again I changed my life. I ensured my consulting days stayed at three days a week. On those days, my staff brought me beautiful cold-pressed juices and healthy lunches and helped to prepare parts of my dinner, like salad or a curry. They also made platters for me for the weekends. I started to book myself in for monthly massages and facials and ensured that I spent my Fridays resting and relaxing. I learnt to say no for the first time in my life.

I realised that I always needed to keep some energy in reserve. I created a great team of staff around me to support my business and lifestyle. I also became an expert in recognising adrenal burnout in my clients and educated them on the signs. I encouraged my clients to maintain balance in their life, and I supported them with herbs and nutrients to maintain their balance. I encouraged regular visits to their GP to keep an eye on their blood pathology, such as iron and thyroid, and warned them that pushing through underlying conditions could also promote adrenal fatigue.

I have then gone on to create programs for my clients and the public on cleanse;nourish; revitalise; and maintain. I also created a program for health practitioners called *I Serve, I Deserve*. My own personal experience of adrenal burnout has led me to truly serve others so they can continue to fulfil their life purpose.

Recently, my son's dad, my ex-husband, was diagnosed with terminal brain cancer. I was grateful that my energy was good, I was not in adrenal burnout, and I had created a supportive team around me. I was able to be by his bedside for his final six weeks, driving four hours back and forth to the hospital. I was once again reminded how important it is that we always keep some energy stored for when our family needs us the most, for natural disasters, or just generally for life.

It is not worth constantly running ourselves on empty until we get to the stage where we have nothing to give. Fill up our own cup first, so that we can truly help others and still be there for our family.

CHAPTER 17

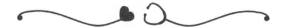

DR ANNE STARK
CONSULTANT PSYCHIATRIST

"I don't know what this is, but it's not a viable pregnancy," said Dr Lyndon, as he frowned in concentration at the ultrasound screen. When I looked at the screen, I saw a grainy, indistinct combination of black and white that was supposed to represent my nine-week pregnancy. I struggled to comprehend what he could see so easily, vainly hoping he had made a mistake. He manoeuvred the vaginal ultrasound probe with the gentle precision of an IVF specialist, yet its cold, hard exterior suddenly felt like an unwanted intruder: an intruder that had stumbled on a truth I did not want to hear. I bit my lip, trying to hold back the tears that threatened to spill from my eyes and draw embarrassing trails down my cheeks.

Having satisfied himself there was no life inside my uterus, Dr Lyndon withdrew the offending ultrasound probe and snapped off his gloves. The familiar sound seemed cold and clinical. "I'm so sorry," he said. "I know how disappointing this must be for both of you. Your first attempt at IVF has not been successful, but you still have six embryos in storage." His face was sympathetic, but sympathy always brought me closer to tears, so I had to look away.

We'll need to book a D and C for this evening," continued Dr Lyndon, as he prepared the consent form for my signature. My shoulders sagged with a mixture of resignation and relief. My exhausted body had been racked with fevers and rigors for the past four days; days in which I had tried to convince myself I had a viral illness. Eventually the lack of other viral symptoms had forced me to acknowledge there was a more sinister cause, even though I'd had no bleeding to suggest a miscarriage.

"What's a D and C?" asked Raf, a frown of confusion creasing his brow as he tried to make sense of the recent turn of events.

I was reminded how difficult it must be for partners of doctors at times like this. My medical training and experience made navigating these situations straightforward, but it was easy for Dr Lyndon and I to forget that my husband had no knowledge of the medical terminology and abbreviations doctors commonly used with each other.

"Dilation and curettage," Dr Lyndon replied. "It's an operation under general anaesthetic to remove the lining of the uterus. We do this for incomplete miscarriages to prevent excessive bleeding and infection. In your wife's case, there is evidence of infection, which the D and C will help to clear."

We were ushered into the waiting room to complete the paperwork required for my surgical procedure. A feeling of dread filled me as the now familiar coldness crept into my body, making me shudder with the onset of another bout of fever. Raf offered me his ubiquitous fleece. It had often been the subject of family jokes, as his English upbringing had taught him to carry one everywhere, even in an Australian summer. Ironically, his fleece made little difference to the cold I was experiencing. Perhaps I was being punished for years of doubting its usefulness. The room began to swim before me as the accompanying dizziness set in, my feverish rigors making it impossible to control my pen.

I reached a point where my stoicism and fear of embarrassment gave in to necessity. I knew if I did not get down on the floor, I would soon lose consciousness and fall from my chair. Feeling ridiculous, I slowly lowered myself to the floor of Dr Lyndon's waiting room. I curled into a foetal position and wished the rough carpet against my cheek would swallow me. I heard the receptionist anxiously making a phone call to request a wheelchair transfer to the emergency department.

In the emergency department, I was asked to undress and put on a hospital gown that was completely inadequate for the cold I was experiencing. It seemed so counterintuitive to take off layers that were keeping me from freezing. On the emergency gurney, I was quickly attached to a blood pressure cuff and pulse oximeter while my temperature was taken. "Forty-two point eight!" the nurse exclaimed, a look of concern on her face as she hurried off to find a doctor. I watched on with a level of detachment as I had an intravenous cannula inserted, remembering how good it felt to palpate the chosen vein and cleanly puncture the skin above to push the cannula through. Being on the receiving end was far less enjoyable. The intravenous antibiotics felt like liquid ice entering my veins.

Gradually my cold abated and I felt a delicious sensation of heat emanating from the gurney under my back. "Is there a heater in this gurney?" I asked a nurse. As if in a dream I heard her speak to my husband over me like I wasn't there, "The heat she feels is her fever breaking. She's probably delirious because her temperature is so high."

I was finally transferred onto the operation table several hours later. My hospital gown and the sheet on my gurney were saturated with my sweat; the fever had finally broken. The anaesthetist began to administer the general anaesthetic. It was a relief to know I would soon be unconscious.

When I regained consciousness in the recovery room after my surgery, I was greeted with a level of concern I was not expecting. Uncomfortable wide bore cannulas in both my arms were attached to bags of intravenous fluid and my blood pressure was being continuously monitored. "We can't seem to get your systolic blood pressure over 70," I was told. "My blood pressure is usually around 110/70," I responded, not yet comprehending the seriousness of the situation.

I was rushed off to ICU, where I was attached to a wall of monitors via a blood pressure cuff, pulse oximeter, ECG leads, and intravenous lines. "It's the infamous Dr Stark," said one of the ICU doctors as he entered, grinning at his private joke. Before I had a chance to ask him why I deserved this title, he told me I was in ICU for treatment of septic shock. "I need to insert a central venous line so we can start an adrenaline infusion to increase your blood pressure," he said. He then launched into an explanation about which central line placements were preferable based on potential scarring. "I think scarring is the least of my worries," I responded. His skilled insertion of the central line was surprisingly less painful than the repeated inflation of the blood pressure cuff on my left arm, which felt like it might fall off at any moment. "We've started you on three intravenous antibiotics," he added.

The following morning, I was startled awake by my mobile phone ringing. I was surprised it had not been switched off. A vague memory that mobiles could interfere with medical equipment surfaced briefly in my mind. Raf handed me my phone and I answered the call in slow motion. I wondered if I was dreaming.

The caller was one of the medical education staff from the hospital where I worked as a psychiatrist. I remembered that I was the junior doctor training supervisor for mental health and was supposed to be in accreditation interviews for our training program that day. The guilty realisation wiped the last traces of sleep from my mind. "I'm so sorry, but I'm in ICU at the moment," I told them. "I'm not sure when I'll be fit to return to work." My comment was met with stunned silence, then a hasty apology as the call was terminated.

At that moment, a nurse walked in and confiscated my mobile. "I'm afraid we'll have to turn that off," she said. "It can interfere with our medical equipment and you're in no fit state to be taking phone calls." Feeling like a chastised child, I was filled with a sense of disbelief. This dream had become my reality.

The days that followed morphed into a nightmare. The bacterial infection that began in my failed pregnancy had spread to my bloodstream and damaged my blood vessels, allowing serous fluid to escape into my body like an invading force. The recalcitrant fluid surrounded and constricted my lungs till I had trouble breathing. It swelled up my legs and abdomen like a bloated carcass that had been in the sea too long. The reduced fluid volume in my blood vessels kept my blood pressure dangerously low. Intermittent pneumatic compression devices on my calves periodically squeezed my leg muscles to prevent blood clots forming.

My mind and muscles ached with the stiffness of perpetual stillness and desperately craved movement. I felt like a fly in a spider's web, imprisoned by an overwhelming network of intravenous and oxygen lines, monitoring equipment, compression devices and a urinary catheter that made it almost impossible to move. I was so nauseous that I vomited up anything I attempted to swallow. I learned the seemingly impossible skill of using a bedpan whilst lying down, as my blood pressure was too low to sit up.

I struggled to accept my newfound helplessness. My independence was an integral part of my self-identity. I was so used to helping others that it felt wrong to be the one in need of medical assistance. In the end, what kept me sane was repeating to myself over and over, "I promise you will never have to go through this again."

I appreciated the distraction afforded by visits from my husband and family, but they clearly struggled with seeing me in the state I was in and had been told to keep their visits brief. I wanted to reassure them that I would be okay, but I knew my words would fail to counteract the visual impact of my current predicament.

After three days in ICU, I was transferred to the medical ward. It was such an immense relief to leave that place of torture, where I had been tied to my bed in the equivalent of four-point restraints. Dr Lyndon informed me I required a blood transfusion, as my haemoglobin was very low. The septicaemia had destroyed many of my red blood cells and damaged my liver. "You gave us quite a scare," he said. "It was touch and go there for a while, but fortunately your kidneys were still working well enough for the diuretics to get rid of the excess fluid."

"Why is this happening to me?" I asked, finally overwhelmed by the gravity of the situation.

"Doctors always get the worst complications," he replied. "That's why we make the worst patients."

I had heard this before and wondered why doctors had that reputation amongst the medical profession. Was it because we were reluctant to seek help for our own medical issues? "Physician, heal thyself," sprang to mind...an ancient proverb attributed to Jesus in the Bible. I had stayed at home with septicaemia for four days before seeking help. I had tried to convince myself I had a viral illness, not wanting to acknowledge the possibility that my first baby had died inside me. My denial had almost cost me my life.

"Septicaemia is a very unusual complication in IVF," Dr Lyndon said. "Would you mind if I presented your case at an upcoming conference, Anne? Completely de-identified, of course." I murmured my assent. If publicising my experience could prevent this happening to someone else, I was happy to oblige.

When I looked in the mirror, I was shocked to see the skeletal frame staring back at me. I had always been thin, but the septicaemia had stolen weight from me that I couldn't afford to lose. My right shoulder began to ache with a deep-seated pain no one could explain. "She hasn't been able to grieve the miscarriage," I overheard a perceptive nurse say to my husband. I knew she was right, but I did not have the strength for grief. All my energy had been channelled into survival.

It was a relief to regain some independence, but my movements remained stiff, slow and cautious. I struggled to lift my right arm and I felt so weak and light-headed that I had to shower sitting down with a nurse assisting me. Despite this, my first shower felt amazing, the soothing warmth of the running water washing away the remains of my ICU experience.

I begged to return home and was eventually discharged. I was told it could take several months to recover fully from septic shock and that I was likely to need an extended period of time off work. I had only been in hospital for eight days, but it felt like a hideous lifetime I wanted to forget.

Although I had left the hospital behind, my septicaemia seemed unwilling to completely relinquish me to the land of the living. It tenaciously clung to my mind and body in the form of nightly fevers and sweats that filled me with fear. For weeks, I shivered uncontrollably in my bed at night and awakened in the early hours of the morning, slick with sweat and an anxiety that clung to me like a parasite. Towels separated me from the comfort of my sheets. A thermometer and a stash of paracetamol took up permanent residence on my bedside table.

I continued to see an infectious diseases physician, but the cause of my persistent pyrexia and night sweats could not be identified. The uncertainty about the origin of my fevers was frightening. Every night in the quiet darkness of our bedroom I imagined the septicaemia reclaiming my body. I couldn't stand the thought of entering that nightmare again – something I had promised myself repeatedly I wouldn't have to endure. My mysterious shoulder pain also decided to linger, making simple tasks such as washing my hair, holding a hair dryer, or even pouring water from a kettle more of a challenge than they had any right to be. The psychiatrist in me was tempted to assume a psychosomatic explanation for these symptoms; the alternative hypothesis of persistent infection was unbearable.

Three weeks after my discharge from hospital, I returned to my work as a public health consultant psychiatrist. I couldn't stand being at home alone with my thoughts any longer and needed the distraction of work. I stubbornly shoved my septic memories into a box buried deep in my mind and my inexplicable pyrexia and shoulder pain finally resolved.

During my first consultant meeting, my executive director joked that my ICU admission was "the most extreme accreditation avoidance" he had ever encountered. I laughed along with everyone else to ease the tension. I was relieved to put that chapter of my life behind me and had no wish to recount the details. As time passed, my recollection of my time in hospital took on a dream-like quality. At times it almost felt like I was a bystander looking on, that it hadn't really happened to me at all.

I attended my first outpatient appointment with Dr Lyndon since my hospital admission. "I feel like I should buy a Lotto ticket," I joked. "Surely I'm due some good luck."

"I think you've used up all your good luck by surviving," he replied, with a wry smile. "If you had come in one day later, Anne, I doubt you'd still be with us." It was a sobering realisation. Even during my darkest moments in ICU, I had not allowed myself to consider the possibility that I might die.

It was three months before Dr Lyndon would allow us to attempt another embryo transfer. "You need to get your strength back," he said. I hated the waiting and counted down the days till we could try again.

"You're a brave lady," my clinical director replied when I informed him of my next embryo transfer date. I was surprised by his comment, as I felt I had no alternative. I desperately wanted to have children, but my career in medicine had consumed me to the point where I had left it too late and now I was paying the price.

I had been inspired by my father to become a doctor from my early childhood. Although he was a GP who clearly loved his profession, he had tried to talk me out of pursuing medicine as a career when I was a teenager. "Medicine is too hard for a girl," he had said. At the time I saw my father's comment as an assumption I wasn't capable of achieving the career in medicine I wanted because of my gender and I was determined to prove him wrong. Now I wondered if he had been trying to spare me the struggle of achieving both my family and career aspirations in a profession designed for men.

Months later, Raf and I were back in Dr Lyndon's rooms hoping for better news. My second embryo transfer had yielded a positive pregnancy test result and I had reached seven weeks gestation. The vaginal ultrasound probe was no longer malevolent, merely uncomfortable. I was cautiously optimistic that this time it would find my baby alive and well. "There's the heartbeat," said Dr Lyndon. "Congratulations!" His facial expression indicated he was pleased to be the bearer of good news this time. I exhaled a sigh of relief. I hadn't realised I was holding my breath. I tried to contain my excitement, as I knew there was still a long way to go, but I couldn't help feeling overjoyed to have this tiny life growing inside me.

When Raf and I met our obstetrician, Dr Renshore, I knew almost immediately he was a good fit for us. He seemed so relaxed and easy-going, the perfect antidote to our understandably heightened anxiety. My attention was immediately drawn to the "No Berthing" sign hanging on the wall above his examination bed. He said a friend had found the sign at a disused marina, but his wry smile revealed his doubts about his friend's explanation. A completely different Mirena provided more humour during our first obstetric visit, as Raf mistook a model of the intrauterine device on Dr Renshore's desk for a fishhook.

At some point during the consultation, my septic shock admission came up. "Ahh, so that was you," Dr Renshore said. "I saw Dr Lyndon's presentation of your case at a conference recently. Quite a few specialists there reported having similar cases, so perhaps the sepsis complication isn't as rare in IVF as we once thought. Let's hope your baby behaves itself this time and doesn't give us any trouble."

Our IVF journey eventually gave Raf and I two gorgeous daughters. By the time our girls were seven and four years old, my traumatic start to motherhood had become a distant memory, although fevers still triggered irrational anxiety within me. My marriage to Raf had not survived, but I knew my love for my girls would expand exponentially over time. The intensity of my feelings for them was like no other love I had experienced and I knew everything I had endured to bring them into the world was a small price to pay for the joy they brought to my life.

I considered myself lucky to have been able to have my first child at 38 years of age and my second at 41. For many women, IVF was a bitterly disappointing experience, full of emotional trauma. I wanted to donate our three remaining embryos, but Raf made it clear he would not consent to this. Eventually, I made the difficult decision to have them destroyed. I cried for weeks afterwards, which no one around me really understood. It seemed like such a loss of potential life that could have given someone a child they desperately wanted. I mourned the lost possibility of having more of my children in the world.

After much self-reflection, I eventually worked up the courage to have a difficult conversation with my father. "Do you remember trying to talk me out of doing medicine when I was a teenager, Dad?" I asked him tentatively. "You told me it was 'too hard for a girl' and I've often wondered what you meant by that."

"Yes, I remember," he replied. "When I was going through med school, women were in the minority, around 10% of the year. They often had to put up with bullying, sexual harassment, and demeaning comments. Women had to be so much tougher than the guys to tolerate that in addition to coping with the academic and work stress of a career in medicine and I didn't want that for you."

Although my father's motivation had been protective, I was grateful my younger self had ignored his advice to pursue a career I now loved as much as he had. The challenges I had faced along the way had made me stronger than I otherwise might have been.

"Medicine is still a difficult career choice for women." I said. "Although 50% of my training cohort was female, most of my consultant colleagues are men. Juggling the study, training and work commitments in medicine with having children can be career limiting for women, especially when they are often expected to take on the majority of the childcare and household responsibilities at home."

"I'm sure that's true," my father replied, "but I'm hoping things are better for you now than they were for female doctors in my day."

"I think women in medicine are more respected now, but I've still encountered discriminatory assumptions and hurtful comments that I doubt my male colleagues have experienced."

I reflected on some workplace incidents that illustrated the disadvantage of being a woman in a profession dominated by men.

Throughout my medical career, I had often dealt with gender-biased assumptions that I was a nurse or a psychologist. I had grown tired of peoples' incredulous reactions when I corrected their misperceptions.

I had been criticised for taking more sick and carer's leave when my girls were both in daycare and our immune systems were frequently battling new viruses. As their mother and a medical professional, it was assumed I would stay at home with our girls when they were sick. I was told I was placing a burden on my colleagues and the health service...as if I hadn't felt that already. A mother's guilt is endless.

I recalled another workplace incident that involved the roller coaster of emotions surrounding my unexpected fourth pregnancy at the age of 45. My initial disbelief had quickly evolved into excitement when I learned of my first naturally conceived pregnancy with my new partner. Bitter disappointment followed when an ultrasound revealed that our embryo had implanted in my left fallopian tube where it could not survive. At nine weeks gestation, I had urgent surgery to remove my ectopic pregnancy before it could rupture. The gestational ages of my ectopic pregnancy and my septic miscarriage were identical, a cruel coincidence that unleashed an unexpected tidal wave of grief I had not dealt with. I hoped my return to work would distract me from my physical and emotional pain. Instead, I was asked to take on additional hours to cover the perinatal mental health service the following week. I was stunned by the insensitive timing of this request.

I found myself wishing there were more women in senior positions within the health sector. Perhaps the current gender imbalance in senior roles was a reflection of women prioritising family commitments over their careers in middle age, as I had done.

Yet, I have no regrets about my choices.

As a mother of young girls, I have developed a growing awareness of the importance of raising them to be strong, independent women with the self-belief they will need to overcome the gender-related challenges they are likely to face in their personal and professional lives.

I am exactly where I am meant to be.

CHAPTER 18

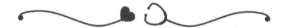

It all hangs in the balance

DR ALISA YOCOM
GENERAL PRACTITIONER

Dear Alisa,

Bon voyage! In a mere revolution of the earth, you'll arrive at the first day of a new chapter in your life. From the airplane seat you're about to become all too comfortable in, you'll descend past the bright morning sun to catch your first glimpse of the endless Australian beaches you once only dreamed about. The bone-chilling minus 20-degree snowstorm that has just farewelled you in Toronto will soon be replaced with the warm embrace of the 30-degree humidity of sunny Brisbane. Don't forget to breathe in that summertime January air. You might wonder what the strange smell is that greets you in the wee hours of the morning – meat pies, of course. Welcome to Australia! But this is no vacation...

Your aspiration to pursue medicine has sent you on a wild ride to Australia. You're packed only with two suitcases, well wishes, and heavy expectations of your success. Embracing the role of an international student, as many others have done before you, to chase your dream of becoming a doctor. For the next four years, you'll be far from family, friends, and the familiarity of home in Canada. This extreme dream-chasing of yours has brought you to the land of sand, surf, and sun...to study? We didn't really think this through, did we?

So, before you stow your tray table and dig into In a *Sunburned Country*, I'd like to ask for a little of your time. Seems easy, doesn't it? Giving away your time. Looking back, I can see that time is the common currency of life. It has no exchange rate. It is priceless. How you divide your time, how you fill your time, and how you make up for time lost will be a constant balancing act. After all, the sands of time flowing through an hourglass must be taken from one side to count towards the other. Each minute of study and each hour spent caring for strangers will inevitably subtract from those intended for your own loved ones. The pivotal moments you will be present for with some patients will echo back your absence for those far away who need you most. It is easy for time to slip away. With it, slowly eroding a space between your two selves. Between you, the 25-year-old young woman, filled with hope and purpose in finally getting to live out your vocation, and me, your 37-year-old self, who is different but the same, made wiser by the hand of time.

You see, I know it wasn't an easy road for you to get here in the first place. I know because I was there. I was there on your first day of university, a young undergrad brimming with hope, when a physics professor asked the auditorium full of biomedical science students, "Who here wants to be a doctor?" Then, in an instant, she threw out the first hit of many to your confidence by continuing, "Well, only one of you will make it." *Maybe I don't have it in me*, you thought.

You discovered the intense competitiveness required to win a coveted spot in a Canadian medical school, heard accounts of students tearing pages from library medical textbooks to thwart their own colleagues. Your caring and quiet nature cowered at the thought of such aggressive self-advancement. You changed majors to biology later that week. *I don't fit the mould*, you thought.

I was there those summers you worked on the assembly line in a car factory to help pay for your university tuition, while others were volunteering overseas to help boost their med school applications. *I'll never stand a chance*, you thought.

I was there when you gave up summer holidays at home to study and sit the entrance exams, only to not receive any interviews. *I'm not good enough*, you thought.

I was there when you applied to med school again after completing a master's degree only to miss out again. *This mustn't be for me,* you thought, and wondered if you'd wasted time chasing an impossible dream.

But there was something inside you that kept the embers burning. This vocation of yours was not going to be on its way anytime soon. Whenever you ventured away to explore other options, medicine called you back again.

I was also there when you finally received that acceptance letter. You did it! You'd been accepted to study medicine...in Australia. But through the joy, the excitement, the relief, came doubt. *Am I good enough?* you wondered, with wavering confidence.

In fact, you're still wondering this as you prepare to take off on your big adventure. Luckily, there has always been someone subtly answering this question along the way with a resounding "yes." Your own little support team, which has been running alongside this marathon with you, ringing that proverbial cowbell with all their might – your parents. A retail manager and a high school grad entrepreneur, Mom and Dad wished for you to have wider opportunities than those granted for them. They always believed you could do anything you put your mind to. They nurtured that belief in you, fostering hard work and dedication in all you did. And, recognising their own parents' oversights in missing their potential career interests, above all they wanted you to find your passion. They knew this would be the key to finding fulfilment for years to come. So, it's no wonder Mom and Dad reacted with all the joy, love, and support, even if it meant farewelling their fiercely independent only child to Australia for four years to study medicine. I see now that your dreams are their dreams, too.

Now this dream that once felt so unachievable, so distant, so impossible, is within reach. Your eyes still blurry from the airport goodbye, your heart knotted in your chest – I know you recognise you wouldn't be where you are without them. This understanding will only grow clearer with every achievement that you will accomplish, and with every challenge and heartache you will endure. The hazy goals of becoming a doctor are finally shifting into focus, even if they look much different than once imagined.

***

You were always a homebody growing up, a child whose best friends were the neighbourhood kids, the kids from your kindergarten class, and primary school – some of whom have been around for decades. You lived in the same home for the first 18 years of your life and went to high school across the road from your primary school. Stability was your middle name. Heck, your grade seven self once hoped you'd get married at the local ski hills and settle in your hometown forever. So, all these years later, when the chance to study medicine in Australia was on offer, suffice it to say it was an enormous leap of faith. And leap you did.

That's what people do when they chase their dreams. They take leaps of faith. And you're about to jump across what feels like a canyon of challenges to get to where I am, with a mere flicker of confidence that you'll make it firm-footed on the other side.

Now, here I stand, on the other side of this earth, from Australia writing to you. To me. I want to tell you it will all be okay. You can do this. You have everything you need within yourself. Spoiler alert – you made it through medical school, you have a career you enjoy, and you even have a family of your own now. It just looks a bit different than you might have pictured.

You always loved a good "choose your own adventure" book, eh? Well, looking back, I've come to remember that you would go back and read all the variations of the story, to make sure the one you chose was the best outcome. There will be moments in your future where you are mentally scouring for some lost pages of alternate endings, some clues to help you choose which storyline to follow.

As your plane slowly taxis towards the unknown, you're thinking you've got the plot line all figured out. You might imagine yourself returning to Canada in four years to train and work as a family doctor in small-town Ontario, perhaps living lakeside with a red canoe, embracing the outdoors as you always have with your family close by. Well, I can tell you there will be twists and turns that change the course of your history and paint a different, at times more challenging, but in many ways more vibrant picture full of love, joy, and fulfilment. A picture that will expand your mind and world in ways you would never imagine. A story that will feature unexpected people, places, and pursuits. I'm here to remind you that in this life, there is no going back to re-read the story of your life with a different ending. In fact, you are the one writing this story.

Our life is the same, you and I. I've just had time to climb some ground for a little perspective. I'm still not very fond of heights, you know. Now, I write to you, to reconcile the choices that will set off tectonic shifts in your life and the lives of those you love. To show you your reflection, a young woman full of potential, capability, and compassion, and have you recognise yourself as the sole writer of this life. While there's no re-writing history, I hope to empower you with the insight and courage to face the challenges you'll encounter, both in and outside of medicine. There's a wavy ride ahead, with much still hanging in the balance for you, but if you trust me, and yourself, will you ever be surprised!

***

If you remember back to a piece of your history, you'll recall learning that for a period of time, Grandpa serviced scales for a living. His experience in keeping things in balance may have saved his life, as his skills were required at home in Canada, sparing him from serving in the war. Were it not for his expertise with equilibrium, there is a chance your entire story might never have been written at all.

Perhaps this partly explains the mesmerising effect of observing the two ends of a balance scale bobbing up and down slowly, finally settling to hover in the air as matching weights perfectly balance the trays. This will be your life's work from here on out. You'll spend much energy trying to figure out how all the study, the stress, the sacrifice can be balanced with all the connections and love you long to grow. The real quest you will embark upon today is to find the balance between your aspirations and matters of the heart.

Studying and practicing medicine is in fact one of the greatest balancing acts you will endure. Right now, I know you're worried about facing the challenges of medical school. A tug of war between determination and doubt. If I could wrestle the shackles of imposter syndrome from you now, I would. It started early for you, with all those initial cracks to your confidence. Yet, paradoxically, the further along you travel in your studies, the higher your qualifications become, the more evidence you'll receive of your competence, the more the beast of imposter syndrome will only deepen the wounds of self-doubt. You will work hard, step out of your comfort zone, and when you do well, the all too familiar thought emerges, *I must have got lucky.* No way, girl. You know who got me to where I am? YOU DID! I'm here to remind you to trust in your ability, be gentle on yourself, and acknowledge your role in shaping your story. Still working on this one, even now, but I at least can see the truth of the matter and how battling with imposter syndrome will help reflect to you your strengths and full potential.

Along this journey, when you trip and lose your balance, remember the friendships and the village of people who will be there to help you back up again. The friendships you leave back home in Canada will scaffold the way forward. Some will stand the test of time and distance and continue to grow, while others will ebb and flow, some fading into the background. You will tirelessly try to keep in touch and connected, making calls, writing emails, video chats, navigating time zones, between study, social, and work commitments. At times, the burden of distance will leave you feeling deflated and heartbroken. *If only they knew how much I missed them,* you'll think. Tell them. They will need you, and you'll need them, too. Never stop reconnecting. These are your lifelines, your soul sisters.

Lucky for you, you are days away from meeting an incredible group of fellow medical students. Among them, you'll find nearly one hundred amazing, adventurous North Americans making the same trip across the Pacific to pursue their dreams of studying medicine. The vast number of applicants vying for limited positions in comparatively tiny intake sizes in Canada meant admissions were dictated by the highest academic cutoffs and extracurricular achievements, leaving perfectly capable, compassionate, charismatic, high-achieving candidates behind. Most, like you, the jewels left unturned by their own medical programs back home. This colliding of worlds with these gems for the next four years will forge friendships that will carry you through your medical training, and some will last a lifetime. You will learn to dance this balancing act together. They will be there when no one else can be. They will understand deeply the sacrifice, the cost, and all the fine print of being an international student. When the heartache of being far from home suddenly storms across the sunny skies of dream chasing, they will be your shelter. When you find it hard to belong in a place where most have roots established, they will be your home. You will work incredibly hard together and celebrate even harder. But as quick as these bonds will form, they will be scattered back across the globe in an instant when med school is done and the next phase of training begins. How proud you will be, though, to be part of this audacious group of esteemed colleagues. Your story wouldn't be the same without them.

***

You won't have any trouble formulating the story of your career choice, though an unexpected detour will be necessary to arrive at your desired destination. I'm sure it won't surprise you to hear that the fast pace of emergency, the intensity of critical care, and the pressure of surgery will not be your cup of tea. You crave conversation, connection, continuity. You are compassionate, curious, and creative. Choosing a specialty will be easy. In fact, general practice will jump out and choose you. You will delight in the sense of belonging you find here, in your desire to keep learning, in the pride you will feel knowing you're making an impact in the lives of others. The surprising part will be arriving at the end of your training pathway, only to become burnt out, disillusioned, and uninspired. The scales will feel utterly out of balance. *This is what I made sacrifices for?* you'll wonder. These will be some of your darkest days of self-reckoning, searching for something that doesn't exist – an alternate ending.

Now, imagine out of the darkness, a hand reaches out for you to hold. To pull you on that detour. A frail hand, her emaciated frame holding within it an expanse of legacy and love. Her time is in short supply. *Who is she?* you might wonder. She will teach you to be present to suffering. She will make you slow down. She will teach you perspective. She will make you re-evaluate. She will teach you to be human. She will transform you. These are the hands of those who will show you the light again. The hands of different souls, a few who are familiar faces in your story, and most of whom you are yet to meet. They will tip the scales back into balance. Pay attention. After all, they hold a special bond with time, the dying.

You will find palliative care crosses your path several times at various stages of your medical studies, career training, and personal life. When you feel lost, you will find yourself again in the many living rooms, kitchens, bedrooms, and verandahs during home visits. You will feel privileged to spend time in the company of individuals, couples, families, and friends, sharing cups of tea, listening to life stories, achievements, and final wishes. Your compassion will shine through in honouring each of them as people, not patients, offering care, kindness, and the dignity they deserve. You will find comfort in the comforting of others on their final journey from this world. You will be deeply humbled and moved by the tragic beauty of humanity at its end.

The colleagues you'll meet in this specialty will be extremely inspirational. They will reignite your joy of medicine and breathe new life into your confidence and purpose. You will see reflections of who you hope to be one day. Your work in palliative care will make you balance time to make it count towards something bigger and brighter. It will remind you who is writing your story once again.

Palliative care will ultimately be the wind in your sail to bring you back to general practice. Once feeling adrift at sea, now safe aground, refreshed with a different set of eyes and ears, a changed heart, and immense gratitude. You will find joy and balance once again in the career you will give so much of your time to. And you will discover that general practice will ultimately give you some of that precious time back in return.

***

Now, let's talk about your greatest fear. You know the one. The fear that is wrenched around your heart as you embark on your journey overseas today. One that will tighten its grip with each visit home, with each subsequent goodbye, with each decision you'll make. The heaviness with which you said your farewells to Mom and Dad, friends and family, especially to your grandparents. *Will I get to see you again?* you'll wonder.

Guilt will grow like a weed in your conscience. For missing those important moments, the milestones, the goodbyes. The airport departure lounge will become an all too familiar vessel of grief, each time with longer hugs, more tears, more uncertainty, more heartache. But unaware, you will grow more strength, more courage, more resilience. You know deep down, as I do now, there will be losses to endure. You will find time when you need to, to revisit, reconnect, and revel in their lives. Remember, you have already made them so proud. The first doctor in the family. Continue to weave the invisible plait that binds you with your elders, as they will always be a part of you and this journey. After all, Nonna and Nonno were migrants themselves, and in fact, this experience will bring you closer to them than you could ever imagine.

As you trench deeper into the marvels of practicing medicine, it won't be hard to suffer more losses along the way. Of relationships. Of your identity. Of belonging. There will be times you'll feel lost in a sea of emotions. Careful, as that metaphor just might play out in real life. But, more to come on this later...

It's okay to feel lost. You will find yourself being pulled between the tides of home and away, only to find that home is becoming smaller on the horizon with each passing year. At times, you will feel like an outsider in Australia, while unexpectedly estranged from your own Canada. Yet, that maple leaf emblazoned on your shirt today will forever be etched on your heart and soul wherever you are. The idea of home will slowly morph away from country, moving instead to moments in time with the people you love.

Your parents, your ever-shining light of love and support, will be there on the other side. You will somehow adapt to living the majority of your family life within the confines of a computer screen or telephone calls. Calendar months and years will turn over, taking with them the milestones, the birthdays, the Mother's Days and Father's Days, and even your beloved Christmases spent apart. But the time spent together will keep you afloat. Those moments you'll hold on to like beacons of hope, so you can find yourself once more and reach a little higher to achieve your goals. And maybe, just maybe, one day you will find a way to all be together again.

***

It's no secret that medicine is a lifelong commitment. There are usually decades of dedication laid down before one emerges a qualified specialist in any given field. It's not surprising, then, that presently, you have already given medicine more attention than any relationship. You will bear witness to the inevitable strain placed on relationships, forcing hands to choose between career and heart. Expectations will erode, temptations will burn, love will waver and crash.

You'll think you have it all planned out now. Be prepared to be surprised. To be caught off guard. To be swept away...quite literally, on a first date in an ocean kayak that will turn your world upside down. Just as the tides can turn, your plans will change. Trust your heart to lead the way to love. Your head can be too focused on what fits, what makes sense, and appeasing everyone else around you. Remember who is writing your story.

Some things may even look like you imagined. You will walk down the aisle amidst family, friends, and lakeside fall colours in Canada. You will look into those eyes and feel embraced by this gentle soul who, in an instant, will make time stop. Those same eyes you first shared glances with, veiled then by the surgical masks and visors across the operating table. The eyes from a world away, yet home. What a story you'll write together.

Some things don't make sense at the time, and it's not until much later one realises that it was all for a greater purpose. There will be a time when you will stop wondering. Much to your surprise, becoming a mother will be the day the penny drops for you. You will look down at that face, asleep in your arms, the tiny hand curled around your fingers, legs folded tenderly against your body. You will feel a heartbeat against your chest that your own will forever drum along with. You will know that every stumbling block, every minute lost, and each difficult decision will have irrefutably led you to this exact moment. To this little person. This perfection. This adventure. The weight of time will be lifted to gracefully and serendipitously sway the scales into balance for evermore.

***

Until then, for the years to come, when you feel the scales tipped in precarious disequilibrium, trust yourself. Hold steady at the helm, realign with your values, and you will balance the ship once more. Reach out when you need to, and you will find the hands to guide you back. Refocus on the bigger picture but delight in the little details along the way. Find time to cherish the important people. Always keep caring, and remember, you are enough. Finally, embrace the art of writing your own story. Now go enjoy the ride, and for god's sake, please always wear a lifejacket!

With love and hugs from Australia,

Me

CHAPTER 19

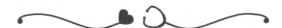

KIM SHEPPARD

NATUROPATH

Mum was slouched in a hoist, hanging from a hospital-grade bed perched in her bedroom, blood spurting from her backside. The wide-eyed look of fear was a tell-tale sign that she had convinced herself that bleeding to death was inevitable...

Her fear slowly subsided as I held a soft paper towel to the ruptured haemorrhoid, reassuring her that death was not occurring today. "We need to move you back to your bed so you are lying flat." One hand pressed the paper towel against the wound to seal the bleed, the other hand using all my strength to lift her hips higher to slow the blood being forced out of her body. Her partner carefully used the mechanical leavers of the hoist to move Mum back over her bed and gently lay her weakened body down onto the bed.

This was one moment in a chain of moments that made me realise I had the ability to powerfully touch, reassure, and motivate people.

Mum was always the light in the room. Her infectious smile and effervescent personality meant everyone knew her. She was the life of any party and always the first one on the dance floor. She encouraged you to join her, with her huge smile and arms outstretched, saying, "Come on, let's dance!" in a playful voice that was hard to say no to.

She loved to rise with the sun to enjoy an early morning run along the Wynnum foreshore. Had a gift for creating tantalizing dishes from whatever she could scramble together from the fridge and pantry. Would stop a stranger on the street to compliment them – and would also tell you where to go if you dared hurt anyone she loved.

It wasn't until she became dependent on her family that I unearthed how unaware she was of how much everyone loved and adored her. Her government department all baked cupcakes for an event they organized, called "Cupcakes for Cass."

"Mum, we have a surprise," I told her. "Your colleagues have raised about one thousand dollars to help pay for your treatment."

Her eyebrows raised in disbelief. Tears welled in her eyes. "I didn't think anyone liked me at work," she trembled.

She loved life and caring for others but still struggled with accepting love and loving herself.

For the fourth time, Mum was diagnosed with cancer and was given a prognosis of six weeks to live. Across 18 years, she had been given the gut-wrenching news that she had cancer three times. As a second-year natural medicine student, I knew this would be the last time.

Mum was not the type of person to make a fuss, and at the time we had no idea how serious her situation was. A tumour had pressed into her spinal column, and over a period of five days, waiting in the emergency rooms of four different hospitals, she gradually lost the ability to walk and became a paraplegic. Her chance of radiation working on day one was 90%, but reduced to 10% on day five. It was unsuccessful.

The tumour on her spine resulted in a complete loss of control of all bodily functions from the chest down due to the progression of many tumours on her right shoulder blade, both lungs, and under her left arm (the size of a grapefruit), which had ulcerated and was oozing through her skin. The intense pain of this disease led her to become a quadraplegic. In hindsight, the paralysis was a blessing. The pain would have been systemic if she could feel the lower half of her body.

As a 23-year-old naturopathic student training to prevent disease and to support people in healing with the abundant gifts of nature, I could not fathom sitting around waiting for her to die, so I deferred a semester and set about trying to save her life. I located a qualified naturopath who specialized in cancer support, and my 6'3" boyfriend would physically carry my strongly built, 5'8" Mum to each appointment.

Mum's partner of 17 years, my brother – 21 months my junior – and myself worked around the clock, making organic meals and juices, measuring countless herbal tinctures, teas, and vitamins, and making fresh homemade paw paw leaf tea that filled the kitchen with a pungent aroma.

I myself have always been fit and healthy with an underlying love for competitive sport. The rigors of representing Queensland in track and field, setting countless records at school, paled in comparison to the hardship and toll of caring for a loved one. It dawned on me that I had finally met my match.

I felt physically exhausted, mentally drained, emotionally wired. Weight was falling off my body, as I was living off vitamins and barely eating. I had chosen to neglect my young, healthy body in a loyal attempt to save my once strong and now frail mum – and best friend.

I attempted to lie on the floor next to Mum whilst she meditated, lying flat on her bed, snuggled in her doona, palms skyward, her closed eyes attempting to block out the pain. On a chilly August morning, through drawn-apart curtains, the sun cast golden rays that warmed her aching body. The garden and trees in her front yard invited birds to sing melodious tunes.

My restless legs and every little sound and niggling sensation became a distraction I couldn't ignore. My mind jumped from one thought to the next. Sitting still for a couple of minutes felt like a distraction from everything I needed to do. I had to keep myself busy to distract from the reality of my situation.

Instead, each night I read Mum inspiring stories. "Women who changed the world: 50 inspiring women who shaped history" left us in awe of women who stood tall and defied the odds to make a difference in the world. We discussed the big questions in life... Why are we here? What is my purpose in life?

"Kimberley," Mum said, "from the moment you were born, I knew you were here for a very important reason. When you were a baby and I was having a rough day, I would just look at you, and you would smile back at me like everything was going to be okay." For the thousandth time she insisted, "You are here for a very important reason, and you are going to be great!"

This wasn't the first time someone had said something similar to me. My acupuncturist growing up, and even random strangers, would say the exact same thing, but I was still confused as to what they meant.

As Mum transitioned to palliative care, I became her daughter again for two weeks instead of her carer. We indulged in sweet caramel tarts and greasy fish and chips from the hospital cafe that left us smiling from ear to ear.

Before entering her drug-induced coma, Mum said to me, "I am going to send you yellow butterflies to let you know when I am around you." My eyes welled as I realised she was not going to be around much longer.

Her days were numbered. Through our meticulous management, we helped her achieve an extra six months to say her goodbyes; speak about those unspoken and emotionally challenging topics; strengthen our already strong connection; bond over our love and fascination of science and the metaphysical world; and discuss the afterlife that Mum was so close to entering.

This journey was a life-defining moment for me.

I knew I could never be the same person again. I had started studying naturopathy to support my future children. To be totally honest, I lacked the confidence that I was smart enough to do this for a living. After embracing this journey and guiding Mum through the final stage of her life, I committed to inspiring people to heal and to make their lives easier. I became obsessed with learning how intricate parts of the body worked. How diet, lifestyle, and herbal medicine can prevent disease and heal chronic illnesses. Staring at my computer during the early hours of the morning became a common occurrence as my fingers typed lengthy assignments. I spent every waking spare moment lying in my yard with my two Staffordshire terriers and my head in a textbook, studying for the next exam, often falling asleep with a book across my chest and my dogs snuggled against my legs.

I threw myself back into study the semester following Mum's passing, not realising at the time that I was dealing with anxiety and depression. My hands were plagued by incessantly itchy eczema, allergies kept my nose constantly irritated and in imminent danger of sneezing; my gut churned with anxiety and poor food choices. Waking unrefreshed from late nights, panic attacks paralysing me, triggered by watching a documentary, left me desperately trying to catch my breath. Heavy and painful periods left me curled up in bed all day whilst still trying to study. I had become so disconnected from myself and was ignoring all the signs from my own body that I needed to take better care of myself. I learnt firsthand how stress and my mental wellbeing could impact my health and how powerful naturopathic medicine can be to heal the body when given the chance.

Seven years later, I graduated with a Bachelor of Health Science as a naturopath with Endeavour College of Natural Health. I married the boyfriend who carried my mum to all of her appointments; by this time, we had an 18-month-old daughter. Things were going well, until I once more found myself in a carer role for someone I loved.

This time, it was my husband.

He had suddenly lost the ability to walk due to excruciating back pain. He writhed with pain and uncontrollable spasms that lasted up to 14 hours for 2.5 weeks until a spinal tap revealed a random streptococcus infection in his spine. Until the infection was discovered, no medications could prevent the pain.

I was working for my family, running my naturopathic business, breastfeeding our daughter, and trying to care for my husband – and desperately trying to convince most of the nurses that my husband was really in pain and not interested in the drugs.

I was broken. Exhausted, standing in the familiar concrete hospital car park, with the strong odour of car fumes wafting around me, head in my hands, eyes red and swollen, completely overwhelmed. I had emotionally hit rock bottom.

I knew that I couldn't keep running on empty. I had done this before without a child depending on me. Something had to change. I had to keep caring for my daughter and my husband. This is what I refer to as my "quantum change" moment in my life.

I realised, "I can only change what is in my control. I need to do things differently so I can keep going."

Once hubby was back at home, set up in his hired hospital bed and slowly on the mend as he learned how to walk again, I found myself needing something for me. It was a struggle to leave the house to shop for groceries without being called home to assist, so I searched for a hobby I could do online. I had stopped working, was a full-time carer again, and needed to do something just for me.

Years earlier, I had become friends with a world famous psychic medium whilst on a spiritual journey to Peru. Passionate about weeding out the charlatans in the industry, she created a certified psychic mediumship school. The idea of going on an internal journey of meditation was inviting, so I signed up for an online beginners course in mediumship that I could do at my own pace.

I transformed a spare room with a laptop, a cozy black lounge lined with colourful cushions, and a throw. A bookcase inherited from Mum was filled with spiritual inspiration. A windowsill to our garden was lined with scented candles and crystals; a Buddha statue sat peacefully on a table beside the couch. On the wall across from the couch hung a picture of Mum and me not long before her illness transformed her body, as well as a canvas reminding me to "Trust your journey." As I relaxed into the plush couch to meditate, I was transported to a place of peace. I had finally found an outlet for all the stress in my life!

During the online course, I found an ability to connect with Spirit. I met some of my Spirit Guides, and during a meditation, I was guided to apply for the first ever Advanced Psychic Mediumship World Summit. My doubts immediately kicked in. *How on earth can I complete an advanced course if I have only just delved into a beginners course?* I needed to apply for this course and answer a series of questions about mediumship to even be accepted. Once I applied, I discovered my experiences from the beginners course had provided me with the knowledge to be accepted into the advanced course.

After nine months of intense training with the Lisa Williams International School of Spiritual Development I earnt the qualification of a certified Advanced Psychic Medium. My passion for meditation had grown, and I could now sit still for over an hour and meditate with ease. One thing that really resonated with me during this course was learning that sometimes healing occurs when someone hears a message from our loved ones who are in Spirit.

I was also shown in my visions and heard, *My purpose is to combine science and spiritualism.* I came out of this meditation wondering what on earth that meant. How can I combine my passion for science with spirituality? Science is evidence based and quantum science was not a respected field of science.

During one of my meditations, I was shown that yoga would support me on my healing journey. As I peacefully came out of the meditation, I contacted a friend, asked for the details of her yoga school, and contacted My Health Yoga immediately. Trusting my intuition, I paid thousands of dollars for the course upfront. Stepping outside to enjoy a cup of tea in my garden and bask in the excitement of embarking on a yoga journey, a yellow butterfly captured my attention! Instantly, my body shivered with goosebumps. I whispered to myself, "Thank you, Mum." A clear sign Mum was guiding me and validating that I was on the right path.

I had only ever completed a few yoga classes at a gym but trusted my intuition and the sign from Mum. I quickly discovered that yoga felt amazing! I was not only releasing physical tension from my body but I was sleeping better, my anxiety had disappeared, and I was healing emotionally. I was learning how to express my feelings by talking about my journey.

As I lay in my sacred room, the air infused with floral scents, I embarked on another meditative journey. I saw visions of Bali. A female Balinese Buddha, sitting peacefully with legs crossed and hands in lap, and the hamsa hand, covered in decorative detail, kept appearing in visions for weeks. I knew I wasn't meant to travel to Bali but that rather there was a connection to Bali.

A few weeks later, I found myself sitting in an old church, which had been converted into a space for hire. The stained-glass windows and high ceilings made the space feel sacred. I was there for a course I had booked months earlier, the Level 1 Australian Bush Flower Essence course. I introduced myself to the lady sitting in the row in front of me. We shared the usual polite introductions and I asked her, "So what do you do?"

To my complete shock, she disclosed, "I have been living in Bali for five years as an energy healer and only arrived back in Australia five days ago." She had been the only form of healthcare on a remote island. When the villagers were fevered, sick and unwell, they turned to her for healing with Australian Bush Flower Essences and Reiki.

My skin shivered and my eyes widened in surprise. I knew I had found my connection to Bali. I instantly felt comfortable and connected with this stranger so I chose to open up to her. "I have been having visions about Bali for weeks."

She was an Australian Bush Flower Essence practitioner and a Reiki Master. I barely knew anything about reiki, but my meditations were guiding me to learn more about it. I shared my visions of Bali with her and mentioned, "When you host your next reiki workshop, let me know and I will be there." I signed up to study reiki with her and quickly found another passion in energy healing!

I made it my priority to fill my own cup with these newfound passions so that I had the physical, mental, emotional, and energetic strength to care for my family. I rose early to start my day with yoga, meditation, and reiki. Eating healthy became a priority, and I made formulated herbal tinctures to care for my gut health and balance my hormones. I even employed my best friend, a personal trainer, to help keep me accountable. I was running my naturopathic business, "Kim Sheppard Health & Wellness," from home and entertaining the idea of how I could pursue my energy practises in a clinical setting.

It was daunting even just thinking about letting the world know I was a naturopath and intuitive. I had always been a people pleaser and had tried to fit in. I was the first in my family to graduate high school and earn a bachelor's degree. I had obtained a science degree even though I had chosen not to study science past grade eight at school. At the time, I felt I wasn't smart enough, and worked hard to prove to myself (and everyone else) that I was.

Now I was considering the possibility of tarnishing this degree by letting the world know I can communicate with Spirit? I had never heard of a naturopath also practising reiki and psychic readings, so I did a quick online search to see if anyone else was brave enough to advertise these services together. I was surprised to see there were a couple, so I thought, why not give it a go. I had trusted every other gut feeling – why not trust this, too?

People started making appointments, and so I travelled to their home or they came to me. I loved being paid to practise naturopathy and energy healing.

I was still caring for my husband and decided I wanted to separate work from home, so I started applying for a naturopathic position at a large clinic. Hubby was still on the mend, so I was looking for a part-time position where I could still be available to care for our daughter.

I scrolled through job sites and spotted a part-time naturopathic position at a large natural therapies clinic and my body confirmed the position was mine. I immediately applied and quickly received a call for a phone interview on the spot. I scheduled a time to meet the directors and practice manager face-to-face.

I was excited. I had let go of any doubt that I wasn't smart enough and knew I needed to step up for my family to provide for them.

A couple of days later, I arrived for my interview at Embrace Life and stepped out of the car to acknowledge a yellow butterfly fluttering past. "Thanks, Mum."

Once inside the clinic, I was greeted with a smile by a receptionist. The walls were painted a calm green with a beautiful tree mural; the floors were an earthy timber lined with green chairs and lush plants, and the air was infused with citrus oils from glowing diffusers, music playing softly in the background. I inhaled deeply and felt my shoulders relax. I felt that familiar feeling, that this was where I was meant to be. I was home. I wanted my patients to be greeted with all of their senses catered for.

Little did I know, I was about to be surprised again. I was greeted by a lady who I had admired 15 years earlier, my manager from my time at Telstra. She had no idea I had applied for the position, as I was now going by my husband's name.

Everything again felt right. I felt comfortable and was myself right, down to the question, "If someone is having a hard time, what would you do?"

I honestly replied, "If it felt appropriate, I would give them a hug." Even though I had been trained to not ever touch a person above the elbow in a professional setting, life and my intuition had taught me to connect with people on a soul level. To treat them like a human, not a condition.

I later discovered five other naturopaths had applied for the same position, but my bubbly personality, inherited from Mum, won them over. I was also offered the position as their yoga teacher.

I moved my business to Embrace Life and found myself working with my intuition during the naturopathic consultations. I tingled with goosebumps as someone shared a childhood memory, a sign to ask, "Did your symptoms first present before or after this experience?" Or I intuitively "ask about their job," to discover that they hate their job, are working 60 hours a week, and have only stayed there for job security. Having always wanted to pursue another path, I asked, "Are you able to start working towards that dream?"

I discovered that my intuition provides me tips to support my clients. I use my science background as a naturopath to ask further questions which validate the intuitive feeling.

During my first year at Embrace Life, a new naturopathic client was hoping for support to conceive after eight years of failure. She had a history that reduced her chances of even being able to conceive by 50%. She was struggling financially, unable to afford IVF, could only afford one naturopathic appointment, and was moving away from Brisbane in a couple of weeks.

My intuition guided me to ask her, "What do you believe in?" She revealed that she was very religious and prayed every single day. My body quivered. This was a unique part of her healing.

I enquired, "Do you pray for yourself, or do you only pray for other people?"

She replied, "I have never prayed for myself. I pray for others to heal and for world peace, but I have never thought to include myself in my prayers."

She could only afford a $20 bottle of flower essences that would last her two weeks to support her fertility, so I also included part of her treatment plan to include herself in her daily prayers.

This was the first time I had included prayer as part of a naturopathic treatment plan. I had rarely prayed in my life, having been raised by an atheist father and a mother raised as a non-practising Catholic who followed a spiritual path in adulthood and chose to be blessed by a Buddhist during her final days of palliative care. I believed what my intuition was guiding me to do.

I was moved to tears when she called from her new home about a month later to happily reveal she was finally pregnant!

Naturopathy was going well, so the next step was to introduce my other services in a clinical setting. I started offering reiki and psychic readings at Embrace Life as well.

I passionately ran workshops certifying people as reiki practitioners and ran spiritual and meditation classes teaching people how to trust their intuition and embark on their own internal healing journey with meditation and intuitive activities. Sharing the importance of trusting their gut instinct.

I realised why I was being guided to learn all of these spiritual practices. I had successfully combined science and spiritualism in a large, natural therapies clinic, supporting people to discover themselves and facilitate their healing journey.

I am so blessed to continue to work as a naturopath and yoga teacher and also regularly practise reiki, psychic mediumship and run workshops and classes that I began all those years ago.

My science background validates my intuitive hits in a clinical setting. I work with people at their own pace, with their own belief systems, to create unique, holistic treatment plans.

I am no longer a people pleaser trying to fit in; rather, I am paving my own path. My own healing journey, my story, is now supporting people with their unique healing journey.

I am proud of myself for defying the odds and noticing all the butterflies Mum sends me. For trusting my intuition, paving my own path, being brave enough to be myself and to support other people to align with their own path and unique healing journey.

I have learnt that healing occurs on many levels: physically, mentally, emotionally, nutritionally, energetically, and spiritually.

People know they need to eat healthy, move their body, go to bed earlier, and take better care of themselves, but no matter how hard they try, sometimes they just can't make this happen.

This is where I can offer extra insight.

I support people in feeling heard. I listen to their stories and spend time with them, asking questions to see how their bodies are handling the various types of stress from their past or daily lives.

I prescribe naturopathic medicines to boost energy levels, regulate the immune system, improve the quality of sleep, reduce pain, balance hormones, and improve gut function so they can absorb more vitamins, minerals, and nutrients.

I provide lifestyle tips, yoga, and meditation to reduce stress and allow patients to reconnect with themselves.

I make flower essences to support them in starting to process the emotions they have suppressed or to channel reiki to balance the energy in the body to reduce stress, pain, anxiety, or to introduce them to their healing Spirit Guides.

I organise various types of testing, including food intolerance testing; or I refer them to their GP, specialists, and other natural therapists to support their health and wellness goals.

I encourage people to unlearn the addiction of busyness and the need to be a super mum who works and studies full time, rushing from one appointment to the next activity.

Personal experience taught me that life has become too busy, overcommitted, and exhausting. My hubby's condition is permanent, and his GP has limited him to working a maximum of eight hours per week, so I continually listen to my body and fill my cup up regularly so I can continue to be a great wife and mother.

My purpose is to help other people to recognise what in their life is contributing to dis-ease or dis-harmony in the body and to provide insight into the physical, chemical, mental, and emotional connections that various types of stress have on the body.

There is a need for emergency medicine, medication, and natural and holistic therapies.

By combining the best of both worlds, clients have a greater chance of healing and discovering the underlying reason as to why they are experiencing their dis-ease.

I recognize that I needed to experience physical, mental, and emotional trauma to be able to relate to my patients. I have walked their path and am proof you can overcome your hardships. I am no different to anyone else. I have provided myself with the time I needed to heal and find my own path.

Their pain may be an important lesson of self love or a story to be told that may help a client, a friend, a loved one, or a stranger to find hope and inspiration in their journey.

I knew I wanted to be involved in evidence-based natural medicine. I didn't plan the rest of it...but am glad I listened to my calling and pursued it!

CHAPTER 20

#make your own door

DR TALAT UPPAL
OBSTETRICIAN AND GYNAECOLOGIST; WHR DIRECTOR

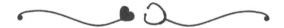

This is my hashtag, my vision and my story.

The wellbeing of women.

Often on a lower priority overall.

Ever since I was a child, I knew I had to work in this disadvantaged space, to try to create some meaningful change, to challenge some norms of cultures and to help break taboos.

Currently, I am an obstetrician and gynaecologist, working in Sydney's Northern Beaches. The picturesque landscape is a bonus.

I grew up in Africa and remember my first day in the Birthing Suite as an eager medical student, feeling immediately that this was what I was put on the planet for. This was my calling.

That passion has remained undiminished, despite the uphillness of some of my journeys and the hoops I have jumped through to get to where I am, to say nothing of the curveballs I have caught and boomeranged!

I migrated to Australia in 1994, and (being the nerd I am) promptly passed all the exams and was offered a training position for women's health which I grabbed with both hands.

I had the joys of three pregnancies during my training to be a specialist, each riddled with hyperemesis. I have done clinical work on shifts with IV fluids running through my veins to resuscitate my dehydrated self. I would cap the cannula to go and see patients, return to the nursing station, connect the IV fluids again, and write up my notes. I recall a professor tapping me on the shoulder during one such episode, with me silently hoping to hear, 'Go home and rest,' only to hear him say, 'You'll be alright, mate,' before leaving the ward to go home himself.

Of all the projects I have helped set up, the most fulfilling remains that of direct outpatient access to IV fluids, in our medical centre, for women suffering from profuse vomiting in pregnancy.

The flashbacks are real, when my patients describe their nausea, and thank goodness I have been able to help women in a similar situation, albeit many years down the track.

It's worth highlighting how incredibly difficult obstetrics and gynaecology training used to be for women who were considering having children during that time; bandaids from family, including my doting parents, made the path easier for me.

Fast forward to 2006, a year special for me as it was when my third child, Tanya, was born; it was also when I became a specialist by being awarded the FRANZCOG title. Years of sweat and sacrifice had come good. I then worked as the Clinical Director of Women's, Children's & Family Health at Manly & Mona Vale Hospitals, in a decade-long role I enjoyed.

For as long as I can remember, I have loved working in teams. I have been an extrovert all my life, at times over sharing; I never really saw myself as a lone specialist in the room, seeing patient after patient all by myself. Nope, that was not my path.

Even worse was the prospect of using my additional sonographic skills, in a dark room, reporting, as a full-time role. Absolutely not. Knowing what you don't want to be or do is also helpful in life, until you figure out the best path for yourself. The one that feels right.

Education is in my DNA, as the child of two gold medalists and university academics, so again, the model of care I sought was to include the role of a clinical educator.

So the dream was something of a combination of all of these, and more.

I decided to call the model 'Women's Health Road', because women are on journeys at different times in their life, with varying needs, and I wanted to try to create a patient-centric care model with a multidisciplinary team holding hands around her. Woman-led care is an even more apt term for what our team eventually designed.

She is an adolescent, wanting support with acne and irregular periods. Then she is a young woman, may want to get pregnant, may not want to get pregnant. Perhaps she has an ovarian cyst now. Has she had an abnormal cervical screening test result? Does she have underlying endometriosis?

Perhaps the menstrual cycles are super heavy. At times, the news is not what we were hoping for, and a malignancy is diagnosed.

Maybe she is pregnant and has a happy, healthy term baby.

Maybe she has a miscarriage.

Then she is perimenopausal: hot flashes, night sweats, mood swings, and vaginal dryness are a concern.

Now she is back with uterine prolapse and urinary incontinence.

Whatever the symptom or need, there should be a structured model of care that can help resolve it. Connected care.

Almost like a one-stop shop.

After I had plotted the 'womb-to-tomb' journey of a woman at different stages of her life, I then identified where we needed support from clinicians with specific expertise or a 'buddy' or 'phone a friend' system. Slowly the team started to come together, because I had worked in the local area for so many years and had many useful contacts and networks, as well as a base of fabulous GPs. My relatively later start into private practice, having initially been a staff specialist until my three children were older, as well as my teaching and training niche and long-standing specific authentic interest in GP education served me well as a solid, supportive referral base when starting out. I had been an OSCE coordinator for the advanced DRANZCOG (diploma program offered by our college of O & G, to assist general practitioners with an interest in women's health to be better set up for real and remote practice as GP obstetricians).

This was a role I had done for a long time, with a superb team; it had given me a wealth of educational and training experience. Looking after a cohort of examiners, both GPs and specialists, with the amazing College staff, exposed me firsthand to the issues relevant to primary care, an experience I enjoyed thoroughly and had learnt so much from.

I feel so privileged to have worked regularly in this capacity, with joint exam co-coordinator Prof Ray Hodgeson (author of *Heartbreak in the Himalayas*). Unfortunately, I was unexpectedly diagnosed with breast cancer and subsequently resigned from this and many other educational commitments. No one in my family has a history of malignancy. I had definitely taken one for the team. However, in my usual stoic manner, I approach this slight inconvenience, a 'nuisance value' problem, with the same can-do attitude.

Lucky was I that I had detected the lump relatively early, before my lymph nodes were involved (results came back clear). I serially went through neoadjuvant chemotherapy, lumpectomy and radiotherapy with much less struggle than I had thought I would,

I think this was due to a combination of:

1. A background of previous hyperemesis, a baseline so awful, with me being in a heap in the hospital pan room on many occasions (my colleagues had suggested they engrave my name on the sink, as a joke). The management of nausea and vomiting whilst having chemotherapy, in contrast, now was so good. I hardly vomited at all, and for me this was a bonus and a constant relief. I am so grateful to my surgeon Dr Kylie Snook for such exceptional care. Being a patient yourself certainly helps your perspective of what you would like women in your care to benefit from, and that compassion is a necessary ingredient in medical management.

2. Having a supportive nuclear family (husband and our wonderful three children), my parents (who helped look after me actively; I did not lose even a kilogram in this journey thanks to Mum's cooking), my sister and her adorable kids meant I was never truly alone.

3. My friends are phenomenal, the type you can truly rely on. Although during my cancer journey I – very unusually for me – did not want to socialise much (though I did attend a number of functions, including weddings etc.). One of my friends created a WhatsApp group for our core circle, a platform for sharing pictures and comments/my feelings at the time. This was therapeutic, and I did not have to repeatedly and individually respond to concerned friends. This now serves as a diary of my malignancy-based journey, which thankfully ended well. I got what is called a 'complete pathologic cure' by having no cancer detected on the histopathologic specimen at the end of chemotherapy. This was a good sign, especially as triple negative cancers can be brutal. Trust me to pick the young brown woman disease!

4. My immediate work family was amazing, I am truly blessed.

This was another reason why I was able to return to my almost normal baseline, so quickly. I accessed the compassion that one should when undergoing treatment. This does not mean that there were not many hoops that I jumped through; not all on this planet are kind and considerate. However, as my personal philosophy has generally been to remain focused on the task at hand, and give less air time to the negative Nancys, so my breast cancer phase too was negotiated with this mindset.

I have digressed. Back to the issue of how my team and I created this unique collaborative care plan for women's health.

My managerial focus was super useful when reviewing the patient care paths through both our service and the supportive interface with the local Northern Beaches hospital, where the women we care for would give birth and be operated on.

It enabled me to partner with a perinatal psychiatrist, a fertility specialist, gynae oncologist, a colorectal surgeon with an interest in perineal tears, a gynaecologist interested in prolapse and urinary incontinence, to enhance our scope of practice.

We have an amazing women's health physio, for on-site sessions, so much value that allied health brings to women's care. Our practice midwife, again adds to the experience and outcome of our patients. I firmly believe that women have a lot to gain from midwifery input, irrespective of the risk status of the pregnancy.

This makes them better prepared for pregnancy and birth in the postnatal period.

I constantly ask myself, what is the differentiating feature of our practice? How can our team create a unique, boutique healthcare medical centre, designed entirely for and by women? How can the patient in our care access the best clinician skillset that they truly need?

Our lived experience does help in providing care, in my opinion. I am often asked by patients if I myself have children etc., and the degree of connection from a firsthand lens is no doubt advantageous, even in the context of some perimenopausal symptoms. Of course, that does not mean that one has to have a clinical condition to care well for a patient. Many of the patients we look after do however, articulate that they would rather be cared for by a female gynaecologist, and that supporting choice for women and our community is a good thing. Our team of clinicians are truly so much like and seem a part of the cohort of women we care for.

The other connection I have felt helped me better meet the needs of CALD women, is my multi-language fluency and cultural sensitivity; being of sub-continent origin at birth and able to speak Urdu, Hindi, and Punjabi means that it is easier to establish trust during the consults.

My firstborn, Mariah Amjad, when helping with the set-up of Women's Health Road, asked if I would consider hiring her friend, Alex Tan, as our receptionist. I was hesitant initially, as I had planned to recruit administrative staff with significant health experience and training.

However I have been blown away by the talent young women possess, too, and the team of digitally savvy front staff has been an absolute joy for us and the patients. They are fast learners and bring a kind of positive, youthful energy that radiates through the building. It has allowed us to innovate with the software companies we chose to use in our practice (clinic to cloud, infomedix etc) primarily because it has a patient portal function, which revolutionised our system and has been a special feature for us. Not only for the convenience of the women and their families that we care for, but also from an ethical environmental perspective. I am so lucky to have a team of like-minded individuals under one roof, wanting minimum paper usage.

From a location perspective, it is an old cottage, located opposite the Northern Beaches Hospital, and next door to a busy GP medical practice, converted into a medical centre after permission from the council, purposefully renovated to serve women during different stages of their lives. So practically easy to care for in patients and emergencies and kind to myself as a clinician. I had no desire to be driving between many hospitals as I see so many of my colleagues do routinely, as my work life balance is important and in my opinion it is better for my patients to access a well rested doctor with a simple routine,

The early pregnancy service in our centre has a separate seating/quiet area, should anyone want more privacy than the main reception. Women who are facing loss or uncertainty of pregnancy outcome can be brought into the service by a separate entrance if they prefer.

The disabled parking is strategically closer with a ramp and a disabled bathroom for the less mobile women of our society.

The menopause service is quite popular; very few such dedicated care models exist, as menopause management overall does not get the resources or attention deserved by such a huge fraction of our population.

The mean age of menopause for Australian-born women is 51 years; the Greek word means the ceasing of menstruation. Women make up 51% of the community. About 80% will experience some degree of symptoms, which for a fifth of women will be severe. This can be a significant quality of life issue. I often wonder, almost on a daily basis, when sitting across women and helping to unpack their symptoms and formulate individualised management plans with them, why they are caring for so many, yet are not caring about themselves. The ageing parents, the teenage children, the partner's issues, job-related stresses and, not to mention, pandemic-related work based impact. It is an endless list that confronts so many women as they pass through mid life.

Are women being heard? We are referred a lot of women with birth trauma due to our structured post natal package. I teach the medical students, 'It is not hard, just listen to what women want,'; our role is to help make complex decision making easier for them, having them in the driving seats of their health journeys. I feel sad when looking after women who feel they were not supported, for example with a timely epidural when they asked for one, or other women who feel they have undergone unnecessary intervention in their past birth(s). We try as a team, when prospectively caring for antenatal women and their families, to value and respect their birthing journey, to encourage birth plans that have been thought through both the experience and the materno-neonatal well being contexts, and to truly understand what matters to them. Whether it is the intrapartum part of their life or a surgical gynaecological journey, for example, the theme is often the same. Anxiety. Desire for solid, evidence-based information. Above all, the need to be heard about their individual preferences. Not to be judged. To be respected. To be well supported when there may be a deviation from what they have hoped for, as childbirth can be unpredictable and it is important for clinicians to strive for the balanced counselling path ie. not to trivialise or magnify risk, as much as possible.

I do love the total continuity of care that private obstetrics offers, journeying with women and their families through such special times is so fulfilling.

Setting up this system has made me understand that medicine is not the only cure, and that the value of collaborative loving care in a safe environment by a multidisciplinary team cannot be underestimated.

A holistic approach, including for example, an additional reflexology session, is what works better for some women. As we have a dedicated psychiatrist, with an interest in the perinatal side as well as a superb midwife with any interest in the psychosocial angle, we have been referred a large proportion of women with mental health based diagnosis, in addition to the gynaecological or obstetric reason. It is our privilege to look after them. To provide coordinated care that is streamlined and structured with a consistent team. Our WHR anaesthetist, Dr Anna Pedersen, has swapped into all our theatre lists providing consistency and comfort of familiarity by getting the women to complete her pre surgical questionnaire whenever possible. This is a unique model of care now, to our knowledge, nationally, with this combination of services and connected method of care delivery, resting on a solid, sophisticated digital foundation.

Our local artist, Michelle Holmes, captured my desire so perfectly in a painting of birds with a heart at the centre that we proudly hang to remind us of the essence of our service to our community.

Organising a private practice has not been a fraction as difficult as I thought it would be. It has been fun and exciting. However, I cannot trivialise some of the challenges faced.

Not everyone you have to interact with has a growth mindset. It is not always easy leading new change.

Medicine can be a territorial space. We are a team of women providing care. As a generalisation, women are often disadvantaged when it comes to leadership and senior positions. This then can expose practitioners to patriarchal cultures, a concept that is getting more spotlight and the attention needed to create better balance for those that come after us.

When I look back at my younger self I realise I blossomed, thanks to my natural interest in education and media, digital health, and management. In addition to the standard clinical role, I was lucky to have been selected for various projects and supported into many positions that then opened more doors for me. However, I was and still am constantly in rooms and forums where I cannot see who I wanted to be. The higher you go, in that context of gender and diversity in leadership, the more you realise that there are some systemic barriers to the success of some groups of our society. Good change is in the air though, with increased conversations and recognition of the value of embracing diversity in all forms, not just the gender based perspective. I am optimistic for the future. I want to be someone who little girls can see and feel confident that they too can achieve their dreams and vision. I am part of the positive change, having the courage to challenge the gaps in the status quo on many an occasion,

Merit is everywhere, but the lens to appreciate it is not always fair. Hence, the title of this chapter/hashtag advice to those that come after us.

Make your own door! Challenge the cultures and traditions that don't feel right for you. These can be in one's personal life (say, with difficult family experiences, marriage-based issues etc.) or more in a professional sense; sometimes the opportunities that are unjustly denied to you or can be the catalyst to look for better paths that, in the long run, were the right ones for you, find the confidence and resilience to search for them. Do not settle for less than your worth. Do not allow anyone to dull your shine. In the end, your talent cannot be diminished by anyone unless you allow that. Have a dog with a bone attitude to creating the present and the future that you want. Make no apologies for this.

Find sources of strength for yourself. I like bush walking, and I enjoy social connections. I am part of a Facebook group with thousands of doctors, 'medical mums and mums to be', with many subgroups and offshoots; it is a part of my identity now. "The hot flush' is a facebook group that focus on connecting and supporting women through the menopause journeys.

In my experience, women are connecting well via social media across physical distances and supporting each other, so seek like-minded groups that you are comfortable in, in which you can be your authentic self. Avoid forums and groups where you feel you are in the 'kateri' court pulpit. Be the change you want to see.

I'd like to end by raising awareness of perimenopause and menopause, as an important transition in women's lives. Too often I see women in your carer mode, juggling ball after ball in the air – except that of your own health and well-being.

You are important. See your GP/specialist, if you are having significant symptoms. There is a lot we can help you with to make this less daunting for you. Reach out for that support, please.

Value yourself.

AUTHORS

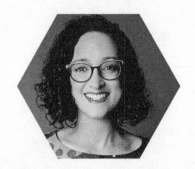

DR ALISA YOCOM

GENERAL PRACTITIONER

MBBS, FRACGP, DipPallMed (Clinical)

Email dralisayocom@gmail.com

Originally hailing from Canada, I moved to Australia to study medicine in 2009 and to my surprise, never left! I graduated from The University of Queensland in 2012 and completed rural General Practice training to obtain FRACGP Fellowship in 2017. I have also obtained the Clinical Diploma in Palliative Medicine as well as the FPAA National Certificate in Reproductive and Sexual Health.

As an adventurer at heart, I remember a GP-lecturer in medical school who likened General Practice to a 'choose your own adventure' career path, and I was hooked. (After reading my chapter, now you'll know why).

I am passionate about all areas of General Practice, especially preventative health and reducing health inequalities. I have special interests in women's health & sexual health, mental health as well as palliative care. I have also enjoyed being involved in the medical education of both medical students and GP registrars.

Outside of medicine, my loves are quite simply, my husband, our beloved son, my family, friends and the great outdoors. It's not always easy finding balance, (especially with a toddler on board), but these are the things that fill my heart so I can continue to do the rewarding job I do.

Creative writing was something I found comforting in my younger years and has always been something I wished to return to one day. Never could I have imagined as a young girl I would return to writing as a doctor, living continents away from my much loved family. To pen an ode to the people who have lit the way along my journey, whilst being indefinitely separated by this pandemic, has been a welcome comfort in itself.

For the young (and not-so-young) folks full of big, bright dreams, this is for you. For international students, for those living in an expat world, or those who feel they have left something behind in return for an immeasurable sense of fulfilment or gratitude, this is for you. And finally, for anyone who has struggled in finding a balance between aspirations and matters of the heart, I hope you will find some words of comfort in my story.

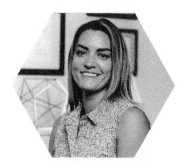

DR ANN MARIE BALKANSKI

MIND COACH & HYPNOTHERAPIST

Email AnnMarie@rapidrealization.com
Facebook @AnnMarieMindCoach
LinkedIn linkedin.com/in/ann-marie-balkanski-md-ccht-b0302556
Website RapidRealization.com

Do you have a purpose in life? I wish I could say I saw mine clearly. It took a very curvy road to find my own path but found it by listening to one thing...myself, or that inner compass guiding me.

I help professionals, executives and leaders clear any blocks to listen and learn about their own inner guidance to discover their purpose and create a clear plan to obtain it.

I am human, I breathe like you and feel like you. I have hurt and cried too but my own unique experiences make me unique as they make you unique.

Being a foster child, high school dropout and getting through medical school, all gave me opportunities to fall down and then learn to stand up faster and stronger. It's all led me here, and I'm writing this now to share what I have learned and done to help both me and my clients to be connected to their higher self. This allows them to live within their purpose by connecting it to the work they do and the life they live. It's an amazing ride to sit in the passenger seat and witness as my clients drive their way to a path of discovery. Maybe there are some bumps and turns but getting to the final destination on the shortest path is what I pride myself in being able to do.

I am a mind coach and trained extensively after medical school on subconscious mind reprogramming techniques. I have a thriving hypnotherapy practice where I see clients one on one and in group settings, both in person and remotely. Prior to becoming a mind coach I was an executive leader for a large network of mental health facilities located throughout the United States of America for eight years. I oversaw the criteria and quality of care of our clients. Educating and guiding professionals, doctors, therapists and mental health facility directors instilled in me a passion and discovery to connect more with what limits us to be our best version of ourselves, allowing us to reach our highest potential.

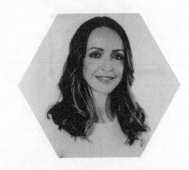

DR ANNE STARK
CONSULTANT PSYCHIATRIST
MBBS, FRANZCP

Email Anne.Stark@health.qld.gov.au
LinkedIn linkedin.com/in/anne-stark-239274aa

I obtained my Medical degree at the University of Queensland in 1998 and my Psychiatry Fellowship in 2009. I have been employed as a Consultant Psychiatrist with Queensland Health since 2010 and I'm currently working at the Royal Brisbane and Women's Hospital. I manage hospital and community patients as well as mentoring junior doctors and psychiatry trainees.

I feel very fortunate to have a career that is intellectually stimulating, emotionally rewarding and allows me to help others. I am also very grateful for the financial independence my career in medicine has given me.

I published a literature review in 2012 and contributed to a published case report in 2021, but have always wanted to revisit the creative writing I enjoyed as a child.

I have two daughters aged 4 and 7, whom I hope to raise in a world with less discrimination and violence against women than I have encountered. I will be encouraging my daughters to pursue their strengths and interests, regardless of whether these are traditionally viewed as masculine or feminine. I wish for them to receive the same respect and remuneration in the workplace as their male colleagues. I hope they successfully manage to navigate the complexities of competing career and family aspirations that are a challenge for so many women.

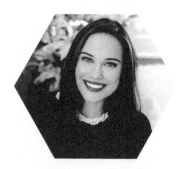

COURTNEY RICKARD

MEDICAL STUDENT, MICROBIOLOGIST, NURSE

Email Hello@CourtneyRickard.com.au
Website CourtneyRickard.com.au

I am a Queensland native with a love of learning, exploring, adventure, and advocacy. I have multiple degrees in health, an MBA, and will soon qualify as a Doctor as I finish my medical degree. My passion is in utilising the combination of qualifications in both industries for improved outcomes for people with barriers in accessing care, whatever those barriers may be.

As a scientist at heart, the type of vulnerable artistic expression required to write a part of one's story is challenging, but I feel there is much to be gained from these stories being told, and being heard.

My experiences have made me appreciate kindness in ways I don't think would be possible were I to have had a "smooth" path. They've taught me that it requires more strength to be gentle than to meet aggression with aggression, and that you won't know what someone else might be traversing if you deduce it by what they present to the world. I've learned to never give up and never stop loving. And that there's nothing more valuable than another human being.

I am ever in awe of my colleagues, grateful for the opportunities to pursue my dreams, and excited about the future.

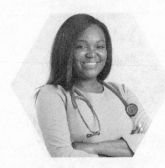

DR ERKEDA DEROUEN

BOARD CERTIFIED FAMILY MEDICINE AND LIFESTYLE
MEDICINE PHYSICIAN

Email elderouen@gmail.com
Website drerkeda.com
LinkedIn linkedin.com/in/erkedaderouenmd

My name is Erkeda DeRouen. As a creative, I get tons of inspiration and ideas to serve communities each day. As a physician, I have taken an oath to help people When I'm not "doctoring" individuals' physical ailments, I am working on impacting others through service and mentorship. I love working to inspire people to be their best selves through one on one interactions, podcasting, and speaking engagements.

I have the ability to connect with the audience in a captivating manner to address a variety of topics ranging from workplace leadership, self-empowerment, health equity, diversity in medicine, and many other hot topics. I have written this chapter to connect with YOU (yes, you) through this book.

After graduating from the illustrious HBCU Hampton University for undergrad, I trained at Boston University School of Medicine, then completed residency at the University of Maryland Family and Community Medicine Residency program. Now, I am working in the healthcare tech sector.

I have been connected to organizations like MIT and Forbes. I will continue to work to inspire and uplift. In my free time, I love spending time with friends and family, traveling to new places, and learning something new each day. I currently reside in the Washington, DC Metro area.

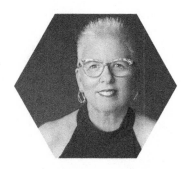

DR FAYE JORDAN

EMERGENCY PHYSICIAN

Email faye.jordan@health.qld.gov.au
Email fjordan@emailcentral.com
Instagram @fayemjordan
Twitter @fayemj63

I came to medicine through a rather circuitous route. As a school leaver, I studied Speech Pathology, pursuing a career in this discipline for almost 20 years, and obtaining a PhD focused on the communication skills of children with acquired brain injury.

In my mid thirties, seeking a "life change", I applied for medical school and the year our eldest commenced grade 1 in school, I commenced medical school. Our second child was born in my final year of medical school. Now, I parent two adult daughters, one a surgical trainee and one hopeful to enter medical school in the coming years.

I am fortunate to work as a Paediatric and General Emergency physician in a busy suburban hospital. My role in emergency medicine offers me the privilege of supporting people on what may well be one of the worst days of their life, and I hope that I contribute to making those experiences a little less daunting.

My husband heads up a successful architectural firm, so life is full and oftentimes challenging. Our home no longer echoes with the sound of children, but rather with the rhythm of adults entering their later years, including my amazing mother who is in her late 90s and still independent.

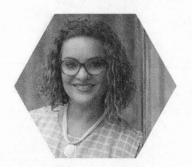

HELEN ZAHOS

BN; MN (EMERG); GRADDIPSCIENCE (PARAMEDIC);
FRSA; MACN

Facebook & Google Helen Zahos
Website helenzahos.com
LinkedIn linkedin.com/in/helen-zahos-74752a53/

I am a motivated, passionate, and caring individual. Over the last 20 years my nursing and paramedical work has exposed me to emergency departments, rural and remote areas, and humanitarian and disaster relief responses. Working closely with different cultures, including Indigenous Australians, refugees, and people seeking asylum. My nursing career has taken me all over the world both on the frontline and on stage, to speak on various issues including mental health for women and chronic health disease in developing nations. I also had the privilege of being invited to be a speaker at a TEDX event.

I grew up on Groote Eylandt, a remote Island in the Gulf of Carpentaria in the Northern Territory of Australia. I completed my nursing and paramedic studies in Darwin, where I was working in the emergency department and was involved with the Royal Darwin Hospital Response to the Bali bombings in 2002.

Since then I have worked in emergency departments in tertiary hospitals; in remote Indigenous communities; attended disaster responses both locally and internationally, and worked with asylum seekers and refugees. My calling is in caring for some of the world's most vulnerable people. I have volunteered in Iraq in internally displaced people's camps outside Mosul in 2017, in Nepal after the devastating earthquake of 2015, and the Philippines after the typhoon of 2013. I also assisted during the Syrian refugee crisis on the border of Greece in 2015 during the height of the refugee crisis.

My volunteer efforts have been recognised internationally for my volunteer humanitarian work, and has been nominated for multiple awards. As 2020 marked the International Year of the Nurse I was appointed the Ambassador for World Youth International's 'Nurses in Action' Program and spent 5 weeks volunteering in Kenya. I am a Fellow of the Royal Society of Arts (FRSA); a Member of the Australian College of Nursing (MACN); The Health and Disaster Management Advisor and founding member to the Commonwealth Business Women's Network (CBWN); The national focal point for Global Networks for Civil Societies on Disaster Risk and the Regional Advisory Group for Disaster Risk Reduction for the Pacific Region; and I sit and advise on a couple of boards for non-government organisations voluntarily.

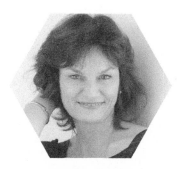

DR HELENA ROSENGREN

SKIN CANCER DOCTOR AND EDUCATOR

MBChB, FRACGP, FACSCM, FSCCA,
MMed, MPHTM, DRCOG

Senior Lecturer James Cook University, Board Member Skin Cancer College Australasia, Accredited GP Supervisor (GMT JCU), Chair Research Committee Skin Cancer College Australasia, Medical Director Skin Repair Skin Cancer Clinic, Medical Director Skinovation Cosmetic Clinic

Email reception@skinrepair.net.au
Website skinrepair.net.au and skinovation.com.au

Having completed medical school and then general practice training in the UK, I came for a working holiday to Australia. One year turned into five and then I found myself on a career path in skin cancer medicine. Seeing gaps locally, I summoned the courage to establish the Skin Repair Skin Cancer Clinic in Townsville in 2009. Boasting sixteen staff the clinic has now completed skin checks for over 22,000 Australians and continues to provide a much needed service for our community.

Ever enthusiastic about my own education, I am a fellow of both the Royal Australian College of General Practice and the Skin Cancer College of Australasia. I have published a number of research papers in medical journals and hold the position as Chair of the Research Committee for the Skin Cancer College of Australasia.

Passionate about upskilling medical colleagues in skin cancer diagnosis and management, I am a senior lecturer at James Cook University, deliver internships at my own clinic for doctors, give lectures throughout Australia and overseas, and was on the working party that developed the Australian skin cancer guidelines published in 2019.

I really enjoy mentoring women to pursue their passions and achieve a work life balance that will enable them to fulfil family and career ambitions while also making a positive impact in their community.

I am enormously grateful for the love and support that my wonderful partner Chris as well as my beautiful mother, son Aaron, and daughter Lydia, continue to shower upon me. You have all made my journey so much more enjoyable.

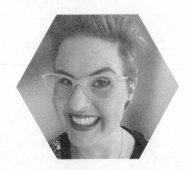

DR JACINTA PALISE

HOSPITAL STAFF SPECIALIST

Raised in a rural town in Central Queensland, I have always been enthusiastic about creative thinking. With an art teacher single mother, I grew up in a house that was always adorned with exquisite colours, fabrics, and sculptures. I was encouraged to pursue poetry and music during my childhood, and was involved in choir, high school musicals, debate team, public speaking, clarinet, tenor saxophone, and recorder. I attended science camps annually in high school including the NYSF in 2004, and studied at the Queensland University of Technology's Conservatorium in September school holidays for clarinet. In this household, there were no wrong ideas, with "failure" seen only as challenges. My mother and brother, as well as my aunts and uncles, really instilled the notions of respect, kindness, and compassion, as well as the need to always try my best.

During my final year of high school, I was involved in a serious car crash, including multiple orthopaedic injuries and a subdural traumatic brain injury. I spent some time in various hospitals, including a rehabilitation unit, before getting discharged home to finish my final term of high school. I hadn't yet been inspired to study medicine...

I then completed an undergraduate dual degree in Arts and Science, then went on to postgraduate medicine, which I completed in 2012. I was encouraged to venture into my current field of medicine by a kind and compassionate clinician who saw my potential and natural skill in his field, and thus began my training. I spent the next few years at various hospitals and community clinics around South East Queensland, where I was fortunate to work with many highly skilled and knowledgeable clinicians who would shape my values and clinical work.

Finishing training in 2019, I have found myself in a regional hospital in Queensland, amongst some wonderful clinicians, a career superimposed on a beautiful, scenic backdrop of coastal bliss. I have founded a local "Women in Healthcare" group and am passionate about driving equality in medicine for minorities, as well as teaching within the hospital setting and educating those in regional and rural settings about the philosophy of patient-centred healthcare.

Mother of one tenacious, wild, and wilful child, I continue to extend on my passion for teaching, currently completing some further university study whilst working full time. In my spare time, I enjoy going to the gym, attending adult dance lessons, spending time with my family, cooking, and kicking ass.

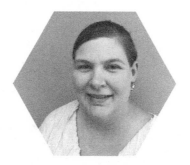

DR JESSICA GEORGE

GENERAL PRACTICE REGISTRAR

Email jessica.george@outlook.com
Instagram @drjessica.george

Before I became a doctor I worked as a Radiation Therapist for several years, providing cancer care to patients requiring radiotherapy after I myself went through life-threatening cancer as a child. I applied and continued to go on to study Medicine at Griffith University in 2007 and worked as an intern in Far North Queensland in 2011.

For me, becoming a doctor was something I could always see myself working towards as I loved not only learning about people and their different journeys, but I have also always loved the progressive professional development and learning required to maintain up to date skills and optimal patient healthcare. Initially I worked within the Royal Australian Air Force as an Aviation Medical Officer. Later, I went on to complete several terms in General Practice under the Royal Australian College of General Practitioners.

Having been a patient myself for much of my childhood, I understood early on just how vulnerable one can feel when you are battling through a life-threatening disease and I have always taken pride in the dignity and honesty with which I treat my patients. No one deserves to be unwell, and I take my role as a doctor very passionately to assist those around me to remain as informed and comfortable as possible, while treating the illness and comorbidities that abate them.

I have achieved so much already in the short period of time I have worked as a doctor, and I cannot wait to see what the next decade of practice will hold. This year has seen the birth of my second child, completing our family, and I look forward to continuing to help each patient I meet to the best of my ability to grow and improve their health and longevity, for comfort and accomplishment that they too can look fondly back upon.

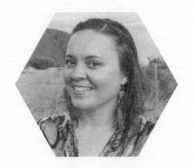

KIM SHEPPARD

KIM SHEPPARD HEALTH & WELLNESS
NATUROPATH

Email looktonature@hotmail.com
Facebook lhwkimberley
Instagram kim_sheppard

Originally from Darwin, Northern Territory, my family moved back to their roots in Brisbane to raise me and my brother. I have always had an interest in health and fitness thanks to my parents. It was no surprise when I started studying naturopathy and yoga. I currently reside in Brisbane with my husband, daughter, two dogs and spend my days pursuing my passions or you will find me out in nature.

Personal and clinical experience has taught me that we need more than a healthy diet and active lifestyle to feel truly healthy. I am passionate about supporting people to find health, wellness, and balance in all areas of their life. To support them to reduce anxiety, overwhelm, and pressure and identify the underlying issues that are contributing to dis-ease or dis-harmony in the body. My passions include fertility, pregnancy, postnatal care, baby and child health, thyroid, gut health, pcos, endometriosis, prostate, headaches, insomnia, eczema, anxiety, allergies, adrenal fatigue, mindfulness, energy healing, intuitive and spiritual mentoring.

I combine my unique skill set to facilitate mind, body, soul healing to support people to find their unique spark in life. Supporting people as they embark on a journey of self-love and self-care to accept themselves for what makes them unique. I also mentor and support other healers to guide them on their journey and to ensure that they are taking care of themselves and prevent burn out.

You can find me at 'Kim Sheppard Health & Wellness' based at:

Embrace Life 4a 4-8 Burke Crescent North Lakes QLD 4509
Naturopath, Yoga Teacher, Reiki Master practitioner & teacher, Crystal healer & teacher, Spiritual teacher & mentor, Flower Essence Practitioner, Psychic Medium

Education – Bachelor of Health Science as a Naturopath - Endeavour College of Natural Health (ECNH), Level 2 Australian Bush Flower Essence Practitioner - ECNH & Australian Bush Flower Essences, Certified Advanced Psychic Medium - Lisa Williams International School of Spiritual Development, Usui Reiki Master - Usui Shiki Ryoho Reiki System of Natural Healing, Level 1 Yoga Teacher - My Health Yoga

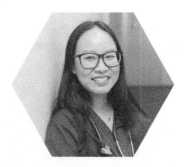

DR LAND PHAN

GENERAL PRACTITIONER
MBBS, FRACGP, DCH

Email landphan@gmail.com

My name is Land Phan – full name 'Thi Hai Land Phan' after my birthplace: Thailand. I arrived in Australia as a tiny refugee from Vietnam just over 30 years ago and although my name and appearance aren't typical – I feel very Australian and am grateful to call Sydney, Australia my hometown.

Being accepted into medicine was a dream come true for an 8 year old who couldn't imagine being anything else. I am proud to say that I completed my Bachelor of Medicine/Bachelor of Surgery degree as one of the first graduates from the University of Western Sydney in 2011, and after that proceeded to complete my internship and residency at the busy Westmead Hospital. I then spent a year furthering my knowledge and interest in Paediatrics at the Children's Hospital at Westmead and obtained my Diploma in Child Health.

I decided that in the end, I loved the whole breadth of medicine and craved the continuity of patient care that a hospital work environment could not give me. I often wondered what became of my patients after they left the wards and couldn't decide which organ in particular to dedicate my life to so I decided to pursue General Practice training and treat whole families. I haven't looked back since!

I am passionate about providing a high standard of care to all families and find it a privilege to be a GP. I am particularly interested in Preventative Health, Antenatal Care, Child Health and Mental Health – sometimes all in the same consultation! I have done further training to provide Focussed Psychological Strategies in CBT and Interpersonal Therapy.

Mental health is an area close to my heart because it's an extremely under-resourced area of need and the effects can transcend generations - both positive and negative. After becoming a new mother myself in 2019, I became even more invested in helping others improve their own psychosocial wellbeing and that of their families. It is never too early to start the conversation about improving mental health and we really need to work harder to reduce the stigma surrounding mental illness in society – particularly in Asian communities and in our own community as doctors.

Healthy doctors = healthy patients.

Writing is my release. I've always written for me, but I started to wonder whether my words could help others as much as I found they helped me. I am excited to share my words with others for the very first time.

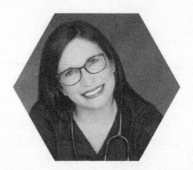

DR MELANIE UNDERWOOD

FACEM; MBBS; BSc
EMERGENCY PHYSICIAN

Email drmelanieunderwood@gmail.com

Pursuing my childhood dream of becoming a doctor, I graduated from the University of Queensland Medical School in 2002.

During the next 10 years I spent my time working in rural, regional, and metropolitan Queensland. I spent 6 months volunteering in Swaziland, Africa before returning to Australia to complete my training with The Australasian College of Emergency Medicine in 2013

I then travelled to Fiji to contribute to the implementation of a new emergency medicine training programme at Fiji National University.

In 2012 I met a fellow emergency physician and together, we had two sensational little girls. Unfortunately when my youngest daughter was only six months old, my partner was diagnosed with an advanced, aggressive cancer and he passed away shortly afterwards.

My unique experiences in life and work have helped shape me into a nurturing, compassionate and dedicated doctor who doesn't just hold a patient's hands during their medical journey, but also holds their heart.

In between raising my gorgeous girls (who are currently 4 and 6) I work part time working in a busy metropolitan emergency department with a focus on teaching medical students and junior doctors. In 2016 I was awarded the prestigious John Pearn Medallion at UQ for Excellence in Medical School teaching. It is my hope that I continue to inspire junior doctors to pursue medical careers in all parts of the world and continue leading a life of passion and hope in the face of any adversity that might come their way.

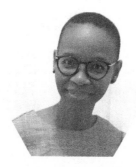

DR MOKGOHLOE TSHABALALA
OBSTETRICIAN & GYNAECOLOGIST
Email mokgohloet@gmail.com
Email info@myobgyn.co.za
Website myobgyn.co.za

I am a 39-year-old Obstetrician and Gynaecologist based in Johannesburg, South Africa. I studied at a then health & science only University called Medunsa, towards my undergraduate degree. I later furthered my studies at the University of Witwatersrand, where I obtained my master's in medicine. I am also a fellow of the College of Medicine of South Africa.

Being an Obstetrician and Gynaecologist affords me the privilege of being part of a family's special journey. From tiny few cells at the beginning to a full human, in a short period of time.

The health and wellness of women of all ages that crosses my path in my Parklane-based private practice is my little contribution to society and the universe at large.

A well woman results in a well family unit. The building blocks of a thriving nation are well families.

When I am not consulting or in theatre operating, I volunteer my time between different, meaningful, and educational causes.

My love for writing began as a 12-year-old girl who wrote in a journal, daily entries for her father who was at the time in a medically induced coma after a car accident. I have not stopped writing since.

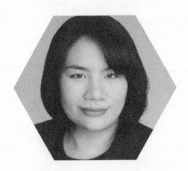

DR OLIVIA ONG

MBBS (Melb), BMedSci, FAFRM (RACP), FFPMANZCA

Email olivia.ong@monashhealth.org
LinkedIn linkedin.com/in/dr-olivia-ong-99814b1bb/

I graduated from the University of Melbourne in 2004. I obtained my Rehabilitation Medicine Fellowship in 2016 and Pain Medicine Fellowship in 2018.

I have a unique story where I sustained a traumatic spinal cord injury in 2008 when I was a pedestrian struck by a car, which left me paralysed from the waist down in a wheelchair. This accident occurred during the early years of my training as a Rehabilitation Medicine registrar. I learnt to walk again after two agonising years, but this experience has taught me to be a more empathetic and compassionate doctor.

I am currently working as a dual trained Physician in Rehabilitation Medicine and Pain Medicine at Monash Health as well as Advance Healthcare Dandenong and Boronia and Melbourne Pain Group.

Through my public and private practice, I empower my patients with the knowledge and medical and holistic pain management treatments to manage their chronic pain, neurological disabilities and/or rehabilitation so they can live fulfilling lives.

I am a Physician Mentor where I mentor junior medical staff at Monash Health and Advance HealthCare. I am also an Educator as I am a committee member of the Learning and Development Committee at the Faculty of Pain Medicine, Australian and New Zealand College of Anaesthetists. I am a Researcher and have published a case report in the Medical Journal of Australia in 2010 which I presented at the World Congress of Neurology in 2012.

In the creative space, I am a Thought Leader in Creative Development and Mindful Self Compassion Practitioner. I am also a Medical Entrepreneur with my creative business 'Dr Olivia Lee Ong - The Heart Centred Doctor', where I am a Medical Leadership Coach, Professional Speaker, Author and Speaker.

My global mission is to help fellow doctors who are suffering from emotional and physical burnout to uncover/discover the benefits of mindful self-compassion and creative development including intuitive techniques, not just for themselves, but for their patients too. My vision is for medical doctors around the world to lead the heart centred lives they truly deserve.

I wrote my Book Chapter to help YOU be aware that your intuition helps you in making all decisions, big or small as it helps you to make CHOICES. This helps you to live a vibrant life in your END RESULT as a CONSCIOUS CREATOR.

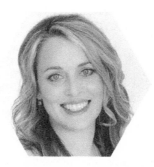

REBECCA LANG
NATUROPATH & NUTRITIONIST

Website healthandhealing.net.au
Clinic Phone (07) 4159 1834

My name is Rebecca Lang and I have a Bachelor in Health Science (Naturopathy) and 3 Advanced Diplomas in Naturopathy; Nutritional Medicine and Western Herbal Medicine. I am not a Medical Doctor. I work extensively with blood pathology and treat with natural medicines. I work to compliment the medical system, encouraging my clients to have regular visits with their medical team. I use natural medicine to safely reduce the side effects of some pharmaceutical medication and also ensure there are no interactions.

I am on the Board of Directors for the Australian Traditional Medicine Society. It is the largest and oldest Naturopathic Association in Australia with nearly 10,000 members. This allows me the opportunity to take my passion for Natural Medicine further and to support its recognition in Australia.

I am a multi-passionate entrepreneur. I own a Naturopathic clinic – Bargara Beach Holistic Health Centre, 4 hours north of Brisbane. I consult in-person for my local community and also via phone and video conferencing for people within Australia and overseas. I created 'Of The Earth Juice Bar & Health Shop' next door to my clinic. This allows me to offer the public cold pressed juices, and gluten – dairy – sugar free vegan snacks and treats, as well as a 3 Day Juice Cleanse.

Recently, I also purchased a publishing business – Of The Earth Publishing. It is currently producing a local magazine going out to 15,000 households every 3 weeks. I also have a Mentoring Program and Internship and support Naturopaths and Nutritionists Australia wide with learning practical business and naturopathic skills.

Over the years, I have had to learn to maintain my energy levels. I am very passionate about my career and what I believe to be my life purpose – a life of helping people. This has led me to become burnt out quite a few times. I have now learnt to recognise this in my clients and teach others about how to find the balance in their life and always keep a reserve of energy for emergency situations.

I have created many programs including 'Cleanse; Nourish; Revitalise and Maintain'. 'I Serve, I Deserve' for health practitioners, and 'Detoxing Your Body, Mind and Spirit'. I also hold regular Detox and Goddess Retreats for women.

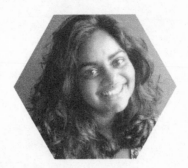

DR SANA JESUDASON
PAEDIATRIC REGISTRAR

This is the bio of a person in flux: I started writing this whilst living in a rental, surrounded by boxes and bags and dismantled furniture that my unbelievably patient boyfriend packed and moved (while I scribbled notes and muttered to myself). I've also recently wrenched all my roots from the ground and moved interstate, bought a new car, started eating meat again and discovered that I am a truly appalling housemate when I'm studying. So fluxy (definitely a word) is my life right now, that in between writing this the first time and editing it the second, I've gone and changed the lot again. Classic Sana.

How I came to medicine is not a unique story. I was raised by doctors (and one badass nurse/midwife), and my sisters are doctors, too. Now, this could have been your typical third-culture-kid, parental-pressure stereotype, but my parents had completely had it with daughters hating med school by the time I turned 17. They begged me to do law or engineering or parrot-keeping, or pretty much anything that didn't involve them listening to another breakdown-via-phone. Nothing else made any sense to me, though; I wasn't sure how I was going to do it, but I knew I had to. I fell in love twice: once with intensive care, and for the second time with paediatric medicine. Halfway through last week, I decided to actually Be happy instead of Aspiring to be happy; I'm going to be a paediatrician, after spending ALL that time and money on critical care exam preparation. Eh. Ya live, ya learn, ya eat some cheese.

I am someone who doesn't do boredom well, so my list of interests is long enough to make me look impossibly indecisive. A curated list would have to start with books, singing and dancing, which are where my soul is happiest, but the one thing I would save in a fire is my miniature tea set collection (yes, all *insert worryingly high number here* of them). I am passionate about fashion that tells a story, and have become an increasingly vocal proponent of pockets as a tool of female empowerment. I am a bundle of contradictions, no more apparent than when I sing jazz harmonies to Slipknot, confusing the hell out of passing motorists. I do not like the nature (because sticky and bugs), but I am reluctantly starting to love bushwalking. Not hiking though. Never hiking, because no.

Contributing to this book means so much to me. I loved writing when I was younger; all oddly sad poems about life experiences I hadn't actually had. Reading back on them, I am vaguely, affectionately embarrassed by how adorably naïve I sounded, how desperate to grow up. I love that these stories, by contrast, are deeply personal: we've all written about experiences that grew or shaped us as medicine women and as humans. I'm proud as punch to be a part of this fantastic group, and I hope you enjoy our stories as much as we've enjoyed putting them on paper.

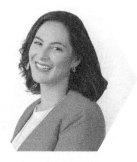

DR SIMONE WATKINS

DOCTORAL STUDENT, PAEDIATRIC ADVANCED TRAINEE
AND PROFESSIONAL TEACHING FELLOW
MBCHB, PGDIPPAEDS, PGCERTCLINED

Email s.watkins@auckland.ac.nz
Instagram @simonewatkinsnz
LinkedIn linkedin.com/in/drsimonewatkins

I am a Paediatric doctor of Samoan descent from Auckland, New Zealand. I was awarded a Chancellor's Award for Top Māori and Pacific Scholar by the University of Auckland to undertake a Bachelor of Medicine and Surgery. I graduated from my medical studies with distinction in 2011. After completing my initial junior doctor years in Whangārei, I moved to Auckland to train in Paediatrics in 2014.

I obtained a Postgraduate Diploma in Child and Adolescent Health and Postgraduate Certificate in Clinical Education and currently co-direct the FRACP written exam teaching course at the University of Auckland. I am currently on a hiatus from clinical work and undertaking a doctorate aiming to find out why the outcomes of critical congenital heart disease in New Zealand differ by ethnicity funded by the Health Research Council (HRC).

I am happily married with two boys, one of which has Achondroplasia, which was diagnosed antenatally. Writing this book chapter has been a dream come true. In the future I wish to continue to advocate for equity, wellbeing, and inclusiveness for all.

The impact that centuries of paternalistic medicine has on women runs deep. There is an urgent need for medicine to improve its engagement of diverse researchers to identify the ingrained biases, including those against women, so we can truly service the needs of society at all levels. This also extends to different racial profiles, socioeconomic backgrounds and disability/ability levels. We have come a long way but there is also some way to go to achieve true equity in the medical world and counter the current inequities.

I hope my story inspires you to be confident and content to be yourself. Only you can define yourself and your future. Life experiences can shape your purpose. You are valuable and important. There is a place for you even if the leaders in your field don't look like you do. Life is a summation of your choices, so choose wisely.

If you want to reach out I am more than happy to be contacted.

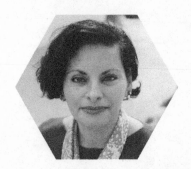

DR TALAT UPPAL

OBSTETRICIAN & GYNAECOLOGIST DIRECTOR, WOMEN'S HEALTH ROAD FRENCH'S FOREST SYDNEY CLINICAL SENIOR LECTURER, UNIVERSITY OF SYDNEY

My daughter asked as a child 'Who is the Disney princess like me?'

As a woman of color, I have constantly been, in forums where I could not see who I wanted to be.

I will be the catalyst of good change in this space, I promised myself.

I am now the Director of Women's Health Road, an innovative integrated multidisciplinary, health care model for women. I am so lucky to work with a phenomenal team to provide holistic care for our community.

Apart from caring for women during pregnancy and birth, our all-female clinician cohort manage a spectrum of gynaecological needs including PCOS, heavy menstrual bleeding, pelvic organ prolapse, urinary incontinence and menopause-based consultations. It is a privilege to support and advocate for women, so many of whom are struggling, especially at midlife.

I am Obstetrician & Gynaecologist working at the Northern Beaches and Hornsby Ku-ringgai Hospitals. My ultrasound training (DDU) is a 'sixth sense' for clinical diagnostic work up. I am also a Clinical Senior lecturer at the Northern Medical School, University of Sydney. I have two administrative based fellowships too. I speak four languages.

My past, decade-long role was based at Manly and Mona Vale Hospitals, as a Senior Staff Specialist/Clinical Director of Women's, Children & Family health.

My educational niche is supporting General Practitioners in the Women's health context. I was the co-ordinator of the Diploma (DRANZCOG) OSCE examination for many years. I am proud to be a media spokesperson for RANZCOG. I am enrolled in a USyd PhD looking at the impact of high-end digital connection with our patients via a patient portal.

I have been privileged to be able to create a safe space for women, that I always wanted to.

Next time you walk into a room, think, are you going to be the change?

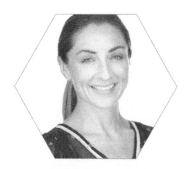

DR VANESSA SAMMONS

NEUROSURGEON, PERIPHERAL NERVE SURGEON
MBBS (Hons) MPhil (Adv Med)
FRACS (Neurosurgery)

Email doctor@drvanessasammons.com.au
Website drvanessasammons.com.au
Instagram @drvanessasammons
Facebook Dr Vanessa Sammons - Neurosurgeon

I am a general neurosurgeon treating all cranial and spinal conditions. My subspecialty is peripheral nerve surgery, treating all nerve compression syndromes, nerve trauma, and nerve tumours.

I think too much, I think. I also probably do too much. I have been asked more than once if I have also 24 hours in a day like people do. I am a neurosurgeon. I have been an engineer, a model, a bartender, a shop assistant. I am also a dancer, a yoga teacher, a traveller, an adventurer, a tinkerer, a skier, a mother, and a weather radar watcher. I love, and I hurt. I have scars, but none that you can see.

I hate excess and anything flashy; you will never see me with a Louis Vuitton bag. But I live in a nice house, with a pool. I drive a German car that costs a lot to service. I live a life of contrasts and sometimes it doesn't make sense. But sometimes life doesn't make sense.

What I do do, is give everything a red hot go. I'll back myself in anything (I genuinely believe that I would be the one left standing if I was in The Hunger Games) and everything I do, I do quite well.

I am a child of a single mother – a nurse and a giver – and I was the first of my family to go to University. I did that, and I never stopped. As a neurosurgeon with a special interest in nerve surgery, I channel my family who have lived before me and I have built on their relatively penniless legacies. All pretty capable and interesting people, but without the means or opportunity. They did what they could, and did it well. I am doing the same.

Am I allowed to count my patients lucky? Well, I do. I am good at what I do, and I treat people as well as I can, and not just for whatever it is that brings them to me.

Being part of this literary project was another thing in this world of things that I do. I enjoyed the freedom of writing about how I am and what I have done in a way that was honest because, if there is anything I have learnt in my years thus far, it is that being honest and raw, acting authentically, that will allow you to find the most happiness, or maybe just contentment, in this world.

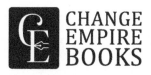

CHANGE EMPIRE BOOKS

WRITE YOUR OWN BOOK

Have you thought about writing a book?

Do you want to raise your profile, get professional speaking engagements, or charge more for your coaching or consulting?

But you're overwhelmed with where to start...?

Maybe you're worried that you're not a good enough writer or concerned what others will think?

You can write a beautiful book, with the right guidance.

Our aim with book coaching is to provide you with all the guidance and support you need to:

- Get clarity on the exact book idea which will position you as an authority and raise your profile so you can attract high calibre clients and/or opportunities.

- Have a clear map of which steps to take each week through the entire writing and publishing process so you never get overwhelmed wondering what to do next.

- Keep accountable to your writing goals so you can set a launch date and stick to it without feeling like this book is taking over your whole life.

- Get feedback to improve your writing each week so you don't have to worry if your book is any good and just know that you're delivering a high quality product.

- Create a strategy for promoting your book so you can be seen in all the right places by the right people, and ultimately, earn more money.

- Have my team take care of editing, formatting and publishing so that you can just focus on writing your book and doing what you do best!

Please visit www.changeempire.com and schedule a free initial chat about your book idea.

I can't wait to hear from you.

Cathryn Mora

Founder, Head Coach and Publishing Director
Change Empire Books

Instagram   @change.empire.book.coaching
LinkedIn   linkedin.com/in/cathryn-mora/
Email   publisher@changeempire.com